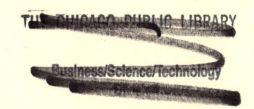

HOSPITALS
What They Are
and
How They Work

I. Donald Snook, Jr.
St. Mary Hospital
Philadelphia, Pennsylvania

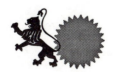

AN ASPEN PUBLICATION®
Aspen Publishers, Inc.
Rockville, Maryland
Royal Tunbridge Wells
1981

Library of Congress Cataloging in Publication Data

Snook, I. Donald.
Hospitals: what they are and how they work.

Includes index.
1. Hospitals. 2. Hospitals--Administration.
3. Hospitals--United States. I. Title [DNLM:
1. Hospitals WX 100 S673h]
RA963.S57   362.1'1'068   80-26956
ISBN: 0-89443-339-3

Library of Congress Catalog Card Number: 80-26956
ISBN: 0-89443-339-3

Printed in the United States of America

Table of Contents

iii

Introduction

Hospitals are among the most complex institutions in our society. They are an integral part of America. Hospitals touch all of our lives. Over the years their basic mission has evolved to the point where they are today the focal point of a community's medical care.

The basic objective of this book is to offer the reader an understanding of the organization, internal operations, and functions of the hospital. In examining the hospital, the book takes a general overview approach. The community general hospital was the model used in most of the book's illustrations and examples. One of the purposes of the work is to acquaint the reader with the methods and systems used within the medium-sized community general hospital. Specifically, the book addresses these questions: How does a hospital function? What are the major components that make up a hospital? Who are the personnel and staff that run the hospital? What are their roles in the organization? Who has the power within the hospital? How does a hospital grow? Where does the hospital fit into the larger medical care system?

The book is divided into several parts that follow a logical sequence. It starts with the hospital's beginning. It then goes inside the hospital, starting with management, followed by a description of the services offered and the departments that provide those services. Next is a discussion of how a hospital is evaluated. The book concludes with some thoughts on how hospitals grow and a description of the elements of a health care system.

Part I

Where Did the Hospital Come From?

A Brief History

THE BEGINNING

It is difficult in the twentieth century to imagine that our modern skyscraper medical centers that serve the health care needs of our sprawling communities really started as something quite different. The word *hospital* comes from the Greek word *hospitium,* a word that is mentioned frequently in the literature from the fifth century A.D. onward. In early history, hospitium meant something quite different from our modern hospital term. Hospitium was a place for the reception of strangers and pilgrims.[1]

In the days following the birth of Christ, Christians were encouraged to make pilgrimages to the many holy places in what is now the Middle East. For several centuries, travelers from Western Europe made their way into this part of the world. Many of these Christian pilgrims traveled without money, believing that they would receive assistance on their way from other accommodating Christians. Many hospitals were established, particularly in more remote and dangerous places. For example, to house the pilgrimaging Christians, it was common for the more well-to-do Christians to bequeath resources in order to provide the travelers with necessary services. These services were extended as tangible gifts in the spirit of Christ. Hospitals were also established by the Christian church as instruments for the propagation of the faith—as living testimonies to the healing mission of Jesus. Many of the great hospitals can be traced to the period directly following the Council of Nicaea in 325 A.D., when the bishops of the church were instructed to go

3

out into every cathedral city in Christendom and start a hospital.[2] The momentum for the founding of hospitiums on the way to the holy city was assumed and aided by several knightly orders that took on the responsibility of establishing and maintaining these wayside places of rest. The best known of these knightly orders was the Knights of St. John, or the Hospitalers.

The oldest hospital in the western world still in existence today is the Hotel Dieu in Paris.[3] This hospital was established around 600 A.D. by Saint Landry, the Bishop of Paris. Even by current standards, this early French hospital could truly be called a medical center, since it embraced many of the varied activities necessary to care for the sick.

Though the Crusades gave impetus to the development of hospitals along the road to the holy land, the travelers brought back to England and other parts of Western Europe the disease of leprosy, which until the time of the Crusades had not been experienced in epidemic proportions in either England or Central Europe. About 1100 A.D., to cope with the spreading leprosy invasion, some 200 hospitals were established in England specially for the care of lepers. This is a large number of hospitals considering that the entire English population at this time was only about three million. These leper hospitals were called "lazar houses."[4]

EARLY AMERICAN HOSPITALS

With the exploration of the New World on the North American continent, various French, Spanish, and English colonies were founded. However, none of these settlements brought about a lasting system of hospitals. Institutions for the sick at that time were simply makeshift arrangements on a temporary basis to care for specific illnesses.

Cortez is credited with establishing the first permanent, solid hospital structure on the North American continent in 1524. The Jesus of Nazareth Hospital is still functioning in Mexico City; it stands as a magnificent example of Spanish architectural genius and a monument to Cortez and the Spanish conquerors of Mexico.

The first American hospitals can be traced to the eighteenth century, well before the American Revolution. These were hastily structured arrangements, built primarily to confine contagious diseases during epidemics. They were founded mainly in seaport towns, such as New York, Philadelphia, Charleston, and Newport. It was not until the eighteenth century that attempts were made to provide continuous service in the form of hospitals. These institutions were called almshouses. They were established primarily for the urban poor and were a direct result of crowding in the urban cities. The first American almshouse was founded in 1713 by William Penn in Philadelphia. It was originally restricted to indigent

Quakers.[5] In 1782, a new building to serve all the urban poor was opened in Philadelphia.

The American voluntary hospital as we now know it began to emerge as a result of efforts of Benjamin Franklin and Dr. Thomas Bond at the Pennsylvania Hospital in Philadelphia. Pennsylvania Hospital, established in 1751, is considered to be the oldest voluntary hospital in the country. Pennsylvania Hospital and the hospitals that followed were established in the same general pattern used for such hospitals in England. Pennsylvania Hospital was built by funds appropriated by the provincial legislature and matched by public subscriptions. The first mental hospital in the United States was constructed in 1772 in Williamsburg, Virginia, and carried the descriptive name of Eastern Lunatic Asylum.[6]

It is important to remember that these early hospitals were devoted generally to the care of the sick, but they were especially used by the homeless and the poor sick. Many physicians did not make use of these hospitals for their private patients. In fact, as late as 1908 the Massachusetts General Hospital in Boston still cared only for the poor, and physicians were not permitted to charge fees to the patients.

The first Catholic hospital in the United States was founded in 1828 by the Daughters of Charity of St. Vincent DePaul in St. Louis. It was called the DePaul Hospital.[7] Some eight years later, the St. Joseph Infirmary was opened in Louisville, Kentucky, as a shelter for orphans and plague victims; it was staffed by the Sisterhood Charity of Nazareth. The reputation of these early American hospitals was not enviable. Because the death rate in these hospitals was staggeringly high due in part to severe epidemics, people considered them their last resort.

The stream of people into our growing urban centers gave a great impetus to the growth of the American hospital. The need for teaching and research facilities led to the establishment of the urban teaching centers and medical school hospitals that continue to be important today in the training of medical students and physicians.

One of the major turning points in the history of hospitals came with the discovery of ether as an anesthetic. The discovery of ether is usually attributed to a Georgia dentist, W. T. G. Morton, who arranged for the first hospital surgical procedure using ether in 1846. Crawford Long later reported that he had used ether during an operation in 1842; however, he did not publish reports of his work until after Morton's discovery was known. The use of ether not only reduced much of the fear of hospitals in the public's mind but also accounted directly for a dramatic increase in surgery that would have been impossible before the discovery.

In the later part of the nineteenth century, following the work of Pasteur in bacteriology and Lister in antiseptic surgery, the hospital began to take on the aura of a place to get well. With the introduction of sulfa drugs in the mid-1930s and penicillin in the 1940s, it became possible to do surgery with considerably less mortality due to infection. From that point on, hospitals began to acquire the appropriate image of a place for citizens to go to receive treatment and to recover.

THE MODERN ERA

Following the close of World War II, American medical technology expanded rapidly. In 1954, the first successful transplantation of a kidney occurred, and with that the modern era of "spare parts" medicine began. Today we continue to experience a modern technological revolution in prosthetic devices such as artificial hearts, heart valves, blood vessels, and the like.

As well as being in the mainstream of medicine's advancing technology, our nation's hospitals are in the middle of an era of intense government involvement. Ever since the Commonwealth of Pennsylvania gave the Pennsylvania Hospital a grant in the 1750s, the government has been assisting our hospitals. Since 1966, when the federal government started paying a significant part of patients' bills with the passage of Medicare and Medicaid legislation, the government's growth in the hospital business has been dramatic. A recent study in one of our large metropolitan areas showed that there were 40 federal agencies, 96 state agencies, 18 city and county agencies, and 10 voluntary and quasipublic groups—a total of 164 agencies—regulating 109 specific functions within our hospitals. Many hospitals are concerned with governmental meddling in the private world of hospitals. Only the future will show whether the hospitals' preoccupation with governmental red tape and bureaucracy will affect patient care.

As we have seen, early American hospitals drew much of their heritage from European hospitals. The institution that we know today as the modern hospital developed quite differently.

Hospitals began to care for the sick almost incidentally. In their earliest forms, hospitals were interested in pilgrims, the indigent, and the plague victims. Later they became institutions where people from all parts of society could come to get well.

Today European hospitals, though quite varied, show many differences when compared to their counterparts in the American system. European hospitals are obviously older but represent a more crystallized system. The government plays a major role in the ownership of European hospitals. In contrast with our Medicare and Medicaid programs, European governments provide much of the financing to European hospitals through social insurance programs or directly from public funds. Planning in European hospital systems tends to be centralized; thus there tends to be a higher number of hospital beds per thousand population than in America. Finally, in Europe the use of outpatient services is extensive, leaving the inpatient hospital to serve the seriously ill. Even the casual observer can see that in many ways America's system tends to be moving toward the European model.

The hospital as an institution has been dynamic; it exists today because it meets the needs of the people. Today's hospitals continue to write history by reacting to the changing needs of society for better technologies of health care and health care delivery.

NOTES

1. Charles V. Letourneau, "History of Hospitals, Part I," *Hospital Management*, March 1959, p. 58.
2. Ibid., p. 59.
3. Ibid., p. 115.
4. Charles V. Letourneau, "History of Hospitals, Part II," *Hospital Management*, April 1959, p. 52.
5. Robin O'Connor, "American Hospitals: The First 200 Years," *Hospitals, JAHA*, January 1, 1976, p. 63.
6. Malcolm MacEachern, *Hospital Organization and Management* (Chicago, Ill.: Physicians' Record Co., 1957), p. 16.
7. O'Connor, "American Hospitals," p. 67.

Chapter 2

Today's Hospital

Key Terms

Types of hospitals ～ *Hill-Burton Program* ～ *Admission rates* ～ *Length of stay* ～ *Patient revenue* ～ *Free care* ～ *Hospital expenditures*

HOW BIG IS THE HOSPITAL INDUSTRY?

There are 7,015 hospitals in the United States. They constitute one of the nation's largest and most complex industries with a total capacity of 1.38 million beds. As a measure of the hospital industry's output, these institutions handled some 37.2 million admissions and more than 263 million outpatient visits in 1978 (Table 2-1). The hospitals had expenditures of more than 79 billion dollars (Table 2-2). The Department of Labor lists some 225 job titles that have a direct relationship to the provision of personal health services. Many of these functions are offered by the hospitals that, in 1978, employed 2.5 million equivalent full-time employees, compared to the total U.S. labor force of 100 million persons.[1]

The hospital industry represents a mix of public and private sectors. Hospitals are generally categorized in one of three ways. First, they may be organized as voluntary (nonprofit) or proprietary (investor-owned for profit). Secondly, they are organized either as general hospitals or specialty hospitals. General hospitals see a wide variety of medical problems. Specialty hospitals limit their care to selective illnesses or patients (for example, a children's hospital). Thirdly, hospitals can be organized as short-term with an average length of stay of three weeks or less or long-term with an average length of stay of a month or longer. Of the total of 7,015 hospitals, 5,581 or 83 percent are community hospitals (Table 2-2). Community hospitals are nonfederal, short-term, general hospitals. Specialty and proprietary hospitals may also be classified as community hospitals. In 1978, proprietary hospitals numbered 732 or 12.5 percent of the total number of commu-

Table 2-1 Vital Statistics of Activity in U.S. Hospitals

	1968	1978
Community Hospitals	5,820	5,851
Other Hospitals	1,317	1,164
Total Hospitals	7,137	7,015
Community Hospital Beds (000s)	806	975
Other Hospital Beds (000s)	857	406
Total Beds (000s)	1,663	1,381
Community Hospital Admissions (000s)	27,276	34,506
Other Hospital Admissions (000s)	2,490	2,737
Total Admissions (000s)	29,766	37,243
Community Hospital Births	3,144,801	3,156,456
Other Hospital Births	105,572	111,975
Total Births	3,250,373	3,268,431
Community Hospital Outpatient Visits (000s)	114,097	201,931
Other Hospital Visits (000s)	42,042	61,675
Total Outpatient Visits (000s)	156,139	263,606

Source: American Hospital Association, *Hospital Statistics,* 1979 ed.

Table 2-2 Number and Types of Hospitals

	Number	% of the Total
Community Hospitals:		
Voluntary (Non-Catholic)*	4,478	64
Voluntary (Catholic)	630	9
Proprietary (Investor-owned)	732	10.5
Non-Community Hospitals	1,175	17
Total Hospitals	7,015	100%

*Includes community hospitals owned by governments. Governmental hospitals consist of both types, community and noncommunity, and total 1,780 state/local; 370 federal. Governmental hospitals, totaling 2,150, account for 30 percent of all hospitals.

Source: American Hospital Association, *Hospital Statistics,* 1979 ed.

nity hospitals. Catholic hospitals, represented by the Catholic Health (Hospital) Association (CHA), are another important segment of the community hospital group. There are 641 Catholic hospitals accounting for 164,403 beds in the United States.[2]

HOW MUCH HAS THE HOSPITAL INDUSTRY GROWN?

There are 975,000 community hospital beds in this country; this is up from the 1969 figure of 826,000. There are 4.5 beds per thousand population in the nation. This ratio has increased considerably since 1946. Outpatient care has also shown considerable growth over the years—from over 156 million outpatient visits to hospitals in 1968 to over 263 million visits in 1978 (Table 2-1). Admissions and patient days per thousand have increased significantly in the last ten years. In 1978, there were 159 admissions and 1,201 patient days per thousand population.

The rapid growth of hospitals in the 1950s and 1960s was an outgrowth of the implementation of the federal government's Hill-Burton Program for hospital construction that started in 1946. This program has been largely responsible for the expansion of bed capacity in the nation. By the end of 1970, the Hill-Burton Program had provided federal funds for the construction of some 336,000 beds; 150,000 of these were in newly constructed facilities, and the remainder were either added, replaced, or remodeled in preexisting facilities.[3] In contrast, non-community hospital beds per thousand population have decreased steadily over the last three decades. For the most part, this decrease is a reflection of changes in medical technology. Significant discoveries have shortened the treatment of many long-term illness conditions, particularly in psychiatric and tuberculosis hospitals.

WHAT KIND OF CARE DOES THE HOSPITAL
INDUSTRY PROVIDE?

Hospitals can be classified into three groups, each representing a special care for the patient. The three groups are psychiatric, long-term general, and short-term (including other specialty community hospitals). Community hospitals account for 975,000 hospital beds or 69 percent of all hospital beds in the country. Community hospitals provide highly intensive care for a wide range of acute disorders. Consequently, they require relatively large numbers of employees for their array of highly sophisticated equipment. Long-term care hospitals, on the other hand, are usually much larger units providing relatively less intensive care for chronic conditions that cannot be corrected as rapidly as acute medical/surgical conditions. As a consequence, the long-term care facilities have fewer employees and usually do not have as many sophisticated diagnostic and therapeutic services and types of equipment as short-term hospitals. Federal hospitals should be excluded from the group that provides general care because they are not ordinarily accessible by the public. Community hospitals represent 83 percent of all hospitals and handle 92 percent of all hospital admissions in the country.

Government hospitals account for 30 percent of all our hospitals and represent a major component in the nation's hospital system. Federal, state, and local governments all own and operate hospitals. Of the 7,015 hospitals in the country, 1,780 are owned by state and local governments. An additional 370 are federal hospitals, including those hospitals serving our military forces. Over the years, government hospitals have assumed a major portion of the burden of providing care for the mentally ill and patients suffering from tuberculosis.

The public's acceptance of the hospital is clearly shown in the growth of admissions between 1939, when 56 persons per thousand population were admitted, and 1978, when 171 persons per thousand were admitted. Due to the reduction in the patient's length of stay from 15.3 days in 1939 to 7.6 days in 1978, the number of patient days per thousand population has increased less dramatically than admissions per thousand.

HOW LONG DO PATIENTS STAY IN THE HOSPITAL?

Patterns of medical practice differ from region to region and state to state. Admission patterns, discharge policies, and utilization review practices within hospitals also differ. The incidence of different types of diseases varies from state to state. Finally, age distributions differ throughout the country and will have an effect on hospital admission practices and length of stay. All of these are variables in the equation of hospital admission rates and length of stay. In less populated areas where residents have to travel long distances for medical care, patients with minor medical conditions might be hospitalized in order to avoid a repeat visit; therefore, shorter lengths of stay will occur in these areas. Economic characteristics, such as income levels in the community and insurance coverage, will also be factors that impact on a patient's length of stay. Hospitals with higher occupancy rates may use an outpatient setting for certain elective surgical procedures. Under these circumstances, the inpatient case mix will be more severe and the length of stay will be greater compared to an average hospital.

The length of stay also differs according to the type of hospital. Patients in state and federal hospitals may stay much longer than those in community hospitals. In 1978, the average length of stay in government hospitals was 8.7 days; the average length of stay in community, not-for-profit hospitals was 7.8 days. The average length of stay for investor-owned (for-profit) hospitals was 6.6 days in the same period. In recent years, the federal government, Blue Cross, and other third party payers have been instituting utilization review procedures geared to restrain the rise of inpatient stays and hospital costs.

WHAT ABOUT HOSPITAL FINANCES?

Annual net patient revenue for all community hospitals has increased from 470 million dollars in 1969 to 55 billion in 1978. On a patient-day basis, gross revenue grew to $219.87 per day in 1978.[4] Occupancy rates increased from 75 percent in 1946 to 80 percent in 1969. In 1978, the rate was down to 73.6 percent. The level of insurance coverage has increased over the last ten years, allowing hospitals a more stable source of revenue. Many hospitals suffer losses due to bad debts and charity care. In such cases, increased insurance coverage has afforded hospitals a more stable cash flow position. There are indications that Medicare programs have contributed significantly to improvements in certain cash flow categories in certain hospitals.

Expenditures in community hospitals totaled 58.2 billion dollars in 1978 (Table 2-3). Labor expenditures—that is, payroll plus employee benefits—accounted for more than one-half of community hospitals' total expenditures. The average hospital employee earned $10,840 in 1978. Capital requirements for the hospital industry are approximately 7 billion dollars per year. The aging of the physical plants constructed in the early Hill-Burton years is putting increasing pressure on the hospital industry's need for capital requirements and capital financing.

HOW MUCH HAVE HOSPITAL COSTS INCREASED?

Hospital expenditures have been rising rapidly over the last several years. They have increased from 19 billion dollars in 1968 to over 79 billion in 1979. Payroll expense, the major component, represents approximately 50 percent of total hospital expenditures (Table 2-3).

Table 2-3 Hospital Costs (Millions)

Community hospitals	
Payroll costs	$28,932
Employee benefits	4,315
Non-labor costs	24,933
Total community hospital costs	$58,180
Total costs other hospitals	21,747
Total costs all hospitals	$79,927

Source: American Hospital Association, *Hospital Statistics,* 1979 ed.

Among the factors contributing to the rise in hospital expenditures are technological changes in medical care and equipment, increased patient demand, and the rising cost of labor and supplies. Most other industries have increased their output by combining improvements in the organization of productive activity with the substitution of capital equipment for labor. However, the hospital industry is a highly intensive labor industry; the substitution of capital equipment for labor is not readily accomplished. Indeed, improvements in medical technology have frequently led to changes not only in the types of cases treated by hospitals but also in methods of treatment that frequently require both more expensive equipment and more highly skilled and technical labor. The public continues to demand more health services to provide this more costly care. This increased public demand over the last two decades has been stimulated by rising consumer income levels, increased insurance coverage, and changes in the demographic characteristics of the population.

NOTES

1. American Hospital Association, *Hospital Statistics* (Chicago, Ill.: American Hospital Association, 1979) p. ix.
2. "Brief Reports," *Hospital Progress,* November 1979, p. 19.
3. U.S. Congress, House of Representatives, Committee on Ways and Means, *Basic Facts on the Health Industry,* 88th Cong., 1971, p. 46.
4. American Hospital Association, *Hospital Statistics,* p. xii.

Part II

Managing the Hospital

Chapter 3

Organization

Key Terms

Classical organizational theory ⁓ Bureaucratic ⁓ Chain of command ⁓ Span of control ⁓ Delegate ⁓ Line ⁓ Staff ⁓ Inservice nursing ⁓ The organization chart ⁓ Chief executive officer ⁓ Assistant administrator ⁓ Functional groupings ⁓ Power

INTRODUCTION

There are two fundamental ways to view a hospital organization. One may look at the overview, or one may consider the departmental organization. Most hospitals in the United States tend to be traditionally organized, that is, they tend to follow the classical theory of organization. The traditional organization structure derives from the theory of bureaucracy developed by the nineteenth century German sociologist Max Weber (1864-1920) and others.

Hospitals are mainly bureaucratic organizations and use bureaucratic principles, such as the division and specialization of labor. Specialization refers to the ways a hospital organizes to identify specific tasks and assign a job description to each person. For example, a nurse's aide has a specific task to perform that is different from that of a physician, a registered nurse, or a medical technologist.

PYRAMID ORGANIZATION

A principle of bureaucratic organizations that applies effectively to hospitals is the grouping of individual positions and clusters of positions into a hierarchy or pyramid. In this arrangement, individuals at the top of the pyramid—for example, department heads—have a specified authority, and this authority is passed down to employees at the lower levels of the pyramid in a chain-of-command fashion. In this way, authority in the hospital is dispersed throughout the organization.

Another effective principle of hospital organization is the consistent system of rules. Hospital rules are really guidelines or official boundaries for actions within the hospital. Examples of such rules are a set of personnel policies outlined in a personnel handbook or written nursing procedures for the care of patients on each nursing unit. Hospitals also use the principle of span of control very effectively. This is especially true in classical functional areas such as housekeeping, dietary, and nursing. Under the concept of span of control, there is a limit to the number of persons a manager can effectively supervise. In a hospital a span of control of between five and ten people in a given functional area is normal to achieve operational effectiveness. Hospitals encourage a pyramid type structure, with supervisors delegating to two or three subordinates who in turn delegate further in a pyramid fashion.

LINE AND STAFF FUNCTIONS

Another important principle of organization that works well in the hospital is the differentiation between line and the staff work. Perhaps the best way to view the difference between line and staff is to regard the line authority in the hospital as connoting direct supervision over subordinates in a direct authority relationship (for example, the head nurse is directly responsible for the work of the employees under that position's supervision). In contrast, the staff function is associated with the advisory activities rather than direct supervision. The delineation between line and staff is dramatically seen in the nursing service department; the line authority is carried out by managers (that is, head nurses, supervisors, assistant directors, and directors), and the educational component (inservice nursing) is an advisory or staff function that supports the line authority.

A TEAM OF THREE

Now that we have examined some of the bureaucratic principles utilized in the classical organization of a hospital, let us take a look at the hospital organization from a different perspective. In A Typical Hospital Organization Chart, Figure 3-1, the governing body of the organization is generally referred to as the board of governors, board of trustees, or board of directors. The board delegates its authority to the administrator, chief executive officer, director, or president of the hospital. At a later point we will examine the various titles of the chief executive officer or CEO. The CEO usually has some flexibility in structuring the administration of the hospital, as shown in the lower half of the organization chart. But again, the same general administrative hierarchical principles apply. The adminis-

Figure 3-1 A Typical Hospital Organization Chart

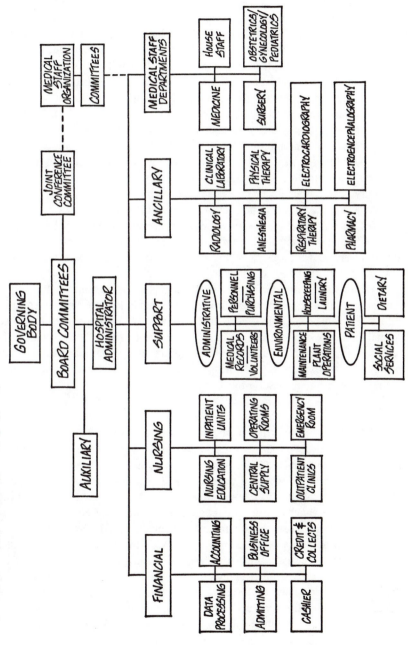

trator generally has associate administrators, assistant administrators, or administrative assistants to handle the various organizational and operational aspects of the day-to-day functioning of the hospital. It is not unusual for an administrator to have support from assistant administrators, the number of whom will vary by hospital size. In very large institutions there may even be someone assigned as "Night Administrator." It is common for hospitals in the 200-300 bed range to have two assistant administrators. Generally this number tends to increase proportionately to the number of beds. It can be seen in the organization chart that the span of control for the administrator and the assistant administrators follows the span of control principle in the classical organization theory.

Below the assistant administrator level in the hospital organization chart, there is a middle management group that becomes the departmental level of management. In the departmental or functional organization of the hospital there are generally at least four major types of functions to be carried out: (1) the nursing functions, (2) the business or fiscal functions, (3) the ancillary or professional services, and (4) the support services. It is not unusual for a hospital to have under the CEO at least four distinct administrative or functional groupings responsible for these areas. Frequently, at this stage of the game the administrators start drawing neat little boxes on their organization charts.

Yet, although an organization chart serves a purpose, in many instances it also has severe limitations. One of the limitations is that it does not show the hospital's informal organization. Also, incidentally, physicians are not shown in any strict formal authority relationships on most organization charts. Though many of the resources of the hospital are often available to the physician in order to meet the physician's and patient's needs, hospitals have not been able to show effectively the resulting relationships on most organizational charts.

One of the reasons that hospitals are so complex lies in the relationships between the three major sources of power: the board, the administrator, and the medical staff. These relationships may be regarded as a kind of three-legged stool or as the tripartite hospital governance concept. Just as the activities of the medical staff impact significantly on the management and governance of the institution, so does the board's action impinge on the doctors. The main organizational units that enable the medical staff to relate formally to the board are the staff's executive committee and the board's joint conference committee. However, the more dynamic links between the board and the medical staff are in the informal day-to-day dealings between the two groups, both in the hospital setting and socially outside the institution. Also, many hospitals have found it beneficial to have one or perhaps two physicians serve as voting members on the board. Thus, there is a team approach to hospital organization. In the classic management or administrative functions we discussed, this approach involves the policy setting and direction of the hospital by the board of trustees. It also involves the principal users of the hospital, the physicians and the patients.

No matter how good an organizational chart might be, the most effective organization starts with the board of trustees and the CEO understanding certain principles of hospital organization. First, they must understand the hospital's objectives. Most hospitals serve patients, and that is their objective. But there are some hospitals, such as university or teaching hospitals, that are also interested in educating medical students and medical residents. There are even a few hospitals that consider clinical research their principal interest. The board of trustees, the CEO, and the physicians must all understand the objective of the institution if it is to be effectively organized. Second, all must understand who is assigned what responsibility. Understanding the players and their roles is important to a successful organization. Finally, hospitals should determine what programs they should offer. Should they offer outpatient programs or detailed inpatient nursing programs?

THE POWER IN THE ORGANIZATION

It is dangerous to generalize about power relationships in American hospitals. Power is defined as synonymous with influence and control. Accordingly, in the hospital organization power can be defined as "any force that results in behavior that would not have occurred if the force had not been present."[1] Beyond this, however, some generalizations might safely be made.

Historically, power in a hospital has rested somewhere between the board of directors, the administrator, and the physicians or medical staff. One observer has noted that "the power of the administrator appeared to be increasing with respect to both trustee groups and the medical staff."[2] The point is that many of the physicians on the medical staff are present (in the hospital) part-time, whereas the administrator has a full-time job in the operation of the institution. The part-time relationship of the physician to the hospital has tended to erode some of the physician's power base. On the other hand, with the tendency in some institutions toward full-time physicians, some power is now being put back into the medical staff, which is having a greater input into many of the hospital's key decisions. U.S. courts have decided that boards of trustees have responsibilities, particularly in quality assurance. The board's fiduciary responsibilities as mandated by the courts have thus brought the trustees into greater involvement with the hospital and given them a greater stake in the power of the institution.

There is no best way to organize a hospital. What works effectively and hopefully efficiently in a hospital is the best way for that hospital. It is clear that hospitals have been rather traditionally organized, which has worked well for the most part. In this context, we might ask if the patients and the consumers will in the future achieve a direction-setting role in hospital organization. With the push for labor unions in some institutions, perhaps traditional management and labor relationships will become more evident in hospital organizations. All of this will be left to the changes of the next decade and beyond.

NOTES

1. David Mechanic, "Sources of Power of Lower Participants in Complex Organizations," *Administrative Science Quarterly,* December 7, 1961, p. 351.
2. W. Richard Scott, "The Medical Staff and the Hospital: An Organizational Perspective," *The Hospital Medical Staff,* November, 1973, p. 35.

Chapter 4

The Governing Body

Key Terms

Volunteer service/Fiduciary responsibility ∾ Consumer representation ∾ Catholic hospitals ∾ Hospital bylaws ∾ Appointing the medical staff ∾ Control of funds ∾ Delegates to the administrator ∾ Medical staff bylaws ∾ Physician's credentials ∾ Darling and Nork cases ∾ Board of trustee committees

INTRODUCTION

As noted earlier, the governing body of the hospital may be called the board of trustees, board of directors, or board of governors. The governing body is responsible for the medical staff's actions, and it hires the administrator. The courts have found that the governing body has to be responsible for all activities within the hospital.[1] Members who serve on the governing body thus clearly have a very weighty responsibility.

The majority of hospitals in the United States fall into the category of voluntary nonprofit hospitals. The voluntary hospital is an integral part of the American way of health care, Since the trustees of a voluntary hospital offer volunteer service and undertake the ultimate responsibilities of managing the assets of the hospital and of setting policy, they assume a fiduciary responsibility. These trustees or voluntary stewards of the nonprofit hospital are private citizens. Although they may be members of some special group or a religious group, they are most often ordinary citizens who simply want to help their neighbors and community.

One of the original reasons for establishing private citizens as hospital trustees was to secure financial support for the institution. By appointing local citizens who had some influence and affluence, the hospital could guarantee a certain amount of contributions to underwrite the care of the poor and the hospital's overall operation. In years past, hospital boards were often appointed so that the hospitals could obtain benefits from their members. Now hospital boards frequently appoint individuals who have particular skills that can help the hospital, for example, with legal advice, accounting assistance, business and management support, or other talents. Today's hospital has a host of legal and accreditation requirements. It is the board of trustees that is required by law to watch over the hospital and its operations.

Hospital trustees serve without pay; they are prohibited from profiting in any way from their membership on the board of trustees. Once appointed, the trustee has a responsibility to safeguard the hospital and its assets. The rewards for being a trustee are the satisfaction of having rendered a service to others in the community and the receipt of some measure of community status by being on the board. Because the trustees represent the ownership of the hospital, they have the ordinary liability of any owners of property. But they have the additional burden of protecting the patients from all foreseeable and preventable harm.

Particularly since Watergate there has been an increased sensitivity to conflicts of interest in our American institutions. As part of a public service establishment, hospital trustees may be vulnerable in matters involving a conflict of interest. Hospitals are coming increasingly under public scrutiny. Some areas, including New York City and Washington, D.C., have prohibited hospital trustees from directly or indirectly doing business with the hospitals in which they serve. More commonly, a state will require that trustees make full public disclosure of their business interests and dealings with the hospitals they represent. Hospitals are well advised to comply to the fullest with the procedures for disclosing conflicts of interest, even though it can be shown in many cases that overlapping trustee interests can actually work to the hospital's benefit, as for example when a trustee gives an institution a favorable loan or expert advice on investments.

WHO ARE TRUSTEES?

As noted earlier, trustees are frequently chosen from among the more prominent members of a community. Highly esteemed businessmen or professionals often serve on hospital boards. It is not uncommon to find representatives of well-established families with inherited wealth serving on boards. A more recent trend, however, has been one of providing community or consumer representation on boards. Yet, on balance, the traditional character of the board still holds. The board's responsibilities are weighty. A citizen's qualifications to be a trustee must be carefully reviewed. Moreover, it takes a while for community leaders to be indoctrinated in the specifics of hospital boardmanship. In a recent survey it was found that governing boards are dominated by business executives, members of the legal and accounting professions, and spokespersons for medicine and hospitals.[2,3]

A special note should be made of hospital boards dominated by religious groups. Frequently, boards of Protestant or Catholic hospitals are dominated by religious groups. Many Catholic hospitals have what might be considered internal governing boards similar to industrial corporations on which the majority of members are sisters. Some time ago, the boards of Protestant hospitals began to include external members of the lay, and today they could be considered to have liberalized their governance. In recent times, many Catholic hospital boards have also been changing; many Catholic hospitals now include lay community leaders as board members.

Over the last decade, there has been a dramatic increase in the number of hospitals that are a part of a formal system or organizational structure. This is a trend that can be expected to continue. Thus, it is necessary to note specifically the role of the trustee in a hospital that is part of a multihospital system. Multihospital systems can include both proprietary (investor-owned) hospital systems and voluntary, not-for-profit systems. Many of the voluntary systems, including a number sponsored by Catholic orders, are religion oriented. In spite of growing centralization, management of individual hospitals usually includes some degree of dual reporting responsibility, first to the local board of trustees, then to the corporate staff. However the local governing body still retains the primary responsibility for the key medical staff relationships. The assumption of a role as a trustee in a multihospital system need not mean the loss of autonomy of the local hospital governing board.

PROFILE OF A HOSPITAL BOARD

Just as hospitals vary considerably in size, purpose, and make-up, so do their boards. A recent survey by the American Hospital Association gives us a good overview of the make-up and structure of the typical hospital board.[4] The average hospital board has 14 trustees, the smaller boards have 8 to 9 members, and the larger boards have around 25 members. Hospital boards typically meet between 10 and 12 times a year; the average is 10. This is reasonable considering a board may not meet during one of the summer months or the Christmas season. Board membership likewise varies considerably. The average term of membership is slightly in excess of 3 years, with a majority of hospitals stipulating no limit on the number of consecutive terms a board member may serve. There is remarkable consistency throughout the nation's hospitals in board committee structure. Perhaps the reason for this consistency is the impetus toward review of hospital bylaws and suggestions from the JCAH. The most common committee is the Executive Committee, which is found in more than 70 percent of hospitals. With regard to the age of a typical board member, over 55 percent fall between the ages of 51 and 70, and 38 percent between the ages of 31 and 50. Over 80 percent of board members have at least a bachelor's degree in education, regardless of hospital size or ownership. Board membership is predominantly male. Across the United States, 83 percent of boards are made up of men, with women representing approximately 16 percent.

FUNCTIONS OF THE BOARD OF TRUSTEES

There are three primary functions or responsibilities of a board of trustees: (1) the formal and legal responsibility for controlling the hospital and assuring the community that the hospital works properly, (2) the responsibility to see that the hospital gains support from its community, and (3) the responsibility of ensuring that the board of trustees is accountable to the citizens and to the community it serves. A board of trustees has a fiduciary responsibility founded upon a trust or confidence. A fiduciary relationship exists when the board has an explicit or implicit obligation to act on behalf of the community's interest.

Specifically, hospital boards of trustees set hospital policies. These policies are general statements or understandings that guide or channel the thinking and action of the medical staff and the administrator in decision making. The governing body has the final responsibility for the quality of medical care in the hospital, the appointment of medical staff members, and the appointment of the hospital administrator.

A review of the activities that hospital boards undertake across the country shows that the following functions can be attributed to them:

- They establish hospital objectives.

- They organize themselves in order to perform their work; this is usually accomplished according to the hospital bylaws.

- They have important roles in reviewing and approving all major plans and programs of the hospital.

- They review all major administrative policies of the hospital.

- They appoint the administrator and evaluate the administrator's activities from year to year.

- They advise the administrator in the operational management of the hospital.

- They review and approve all major hospital decisions.

- They annually review the hospital's performance to see whether the hospital has reached its objectives.

The board's important role in the control of hospital funds should be noted. It is the board's responsibility to see that the hospital's finances be reviewed in some detail and approved by the trustees. Hopefully, most governing board members will be involved in obtaining endowments, grants, gifts, and other donation income. If the hospital is fortunate enough to have a significant amount of funds to be invested, it is the hospital board's responsibility to do this. Frequently, this is done at least once a year at the time the hospital budget is presented to the board of trustees by the hospital administrator. The hospital has an annual audit by a public accounting firm in order to see that these funds have been expended and accounted for properly. This audit is reported to the hospital board of trustees.

HIRING THE ADMINISTRATOR

To assist the board of trustees in managing the hospital, the trustees have an obligation to hire a competent hospital administrator to oversee the day-to-day management of the hospital activities. One of the most important functions of a board of trustees is the investigation, review, and selection of the hospital adminis-trator. Indeed, perhaps the most important thing a board of trustees does is to select an administrator. Hospitals are big business, and trustees must seek executives who have strengths in planning, organizing, and controlling, as well as proven leadership skills. The board then delegates to the administrator the authority and responsibility to manage the day-to-day operations of the hospital. However, though the trustees must delegate enough authority so that the administrator can do this job well, the board still retains the ultimate responsibility for everything that happens in the hospital. The relationship between the administrator and the governing board is primarily that of employee-employer, but not in the usual sense of the term. Since the hospital is a very special type of organization, the relation-ship between the administrator and the governing board is in fact similar to a partnership. Just as it is the responsibility of the governing boards to hire adminis-trators, it is also their responsibility to discharge them for cause at any time.

RELATIONSHIP WITH THE MEDICAL STAFF

The medical staff of the hospital operates within its own medical staff bylaws and regulations, but the physicians on the medical staff are accountable to the board of trustees for the professional care of their patients. The board of trustees is responsible for exercising due care in the selection of physicians. A physician's application credentials and requested privileges are carefully examined by the medical staff, which in turn recommends the physician with requested privileges to the board. It is the responsibility of the trustees to act upon these recommendations, that is, to grant privileges, to request further clarification from the medical staff, or to reject the privileges on sound grounds. Although to the layman it may seem strange that the board of trustees has the ultimate decision as to the physician's rights and privileges to practice in the hospital, the board must in fact be fully competent to review the traits and past history of the hospital's physicians.

One of the more important elements of a trustee's job has been reviewed in some detail by the courts, namely, the trustee's responsibility for quality care. In effect, the board of trustees is legally responsible for the care rendered by the hospital's employees and attending physicians. Indeed, court decisions have indicated that the board of trustees has a duty that may go beyond simple delegation of authority to the medical staff and accepting the medical staff's recommendations. In the hallmark *Darling* case *(Darling v. Charleston Community Memorial Hospital, 1965)*, the courts ruled for the plaintiff, who was a patient, and held that the hospital corporation was liable because it did not intervene, through its employee administrator and nurses, to prevent a damage that had occurred through the negligence of one of the hospital's attending physicians.[5]

Following the *Darling* case, the courts, in 1973, again found, in the case of *Gonzales v. Mercy General Hospital in Sacramento, California, and John J. Nork, M.D.*, that a hospital, by virtue of its custody of the patient, owes the patient a duty of care.[6] The court noted that Dr. Nork had performed 36 unnecessary operations over a nine-year period. The court found that the board of trustees has an obligation to purge the hospital of inadequate physicians. This duty includes the obligation to protect the patient from acts of malpractice by an independently retained physician who is a member of the hospital's medical staff. The court further indicated that if the hospital knows, has reason to know, or should know that negligent acts are likely to occur, it has a responsibility to protect the patient. Even if the board members fail to understand this, the courts have indicated very strongly and very clearly that it is the trustees who have the corporate responsibility for the quality of care in our hospitals. It is now recognized that a board of trustees cannot delegate this responsibility; it can only delegate authority in assigned functions.

Thus, the board of trustees has a legal and moral responsibility to control the quality of medical care in the hospital. Yet, though the governing body has the ultimate responsibility, quality control is a team effort. The CEO and the chief of the medical staff also have a part to play in the quality assurance program. Such a program has to be developed and implemented, and both the administrator and chief of the medical staff contribute greatly in these two areas. The board has the monitoring role in the program. Monitoring includes receiving monthly reports that display the medical staff's performance as measured against preestablished criteria, concurring with medical staff recommendations, or developing the board's own recommendations to improve medical staff performance and to ensure that it impacts positively on the quality of medical care.

The typical board of trustees delegates to the medical staff the day-to-day medical affairs of the hospital. In most things, the medical staff functions autonomously as a self-governing body. The board's joint conference committee, which has representatives from the medical staff, serves as the main formal linkage between the medical arm of the hospital and the board and its administrator.

HOW DOES THE BOARD OPERATE?

The board of trustees operates under the bylaws of the hospital. The bylaws spell out how a hospital board is founded and how it operates to attain its objectives. Typical bylaws include a statement on the hospital's purpose and the responsibilities of the board. It also contains a statement of authority for the board to appoint the administrator and the medical staff. In addition, the bylaws outline how board members are appointed and for what period of time. Most bylaws indicate an elaborate committee structure. It is through these committees that the governing board usually gets its work accomplished. This committee structure is frequently established along special functional lines. Examples of typical board of trustee committees are an executive committee, a finance committee, a planning committee, and perhaps a committee for the building and its operations and grounds. Generally, recommendations through the separate committees affect the governance, management, and administration, as well as the medical staff in the hospital.

It is the duty of the board to select carefully the members of these board committees. The caliber of the recommendations that emerge from these committees, and subsequently the caliber of the resulting board action, is frequently a function of the quality of selection that went into the committee assignments. The administrator, through the application of leadership skills and management delegation, and in close relationship with these board committees, frequently provides the ultimate key to success in all aspects of the hospital operation.

NOTES

1. Robert M. Cunningham, Jr., *Governing Hospitals: Trustees and the New Accountabilities* (Chicago, Ill.: American Hospital Association, 1976), p. 32.
2. Anthony R. Kovener, "Governing Boards," *Hospital Administration*, Winter 1975, p. 67.
3. Rockwell Schulz and Alton C. Johnson, *Management of Hospitals* (New York, N.Y.: McGraw-Hill Book Co., 1976), p. 51.
4. Gregory J. Nigosian, "New Data on Hospital Governing Boards," *Trustee*, September 1980, pp. 18-25.
5. *Darling v. Charleston Community Memorial Hospital*, 211 N.E. 2d 253 (1965) cert. denied 383 V.S. 946 (1966).
6. Cunningham, *Governing Hospitals*, p. 80.

Chapter 5

The Hospital Administrator

Key Terms

Chief executive officer (CEO) ~ *American College of Hospital Administrators (ACHA)* ~ *Internal operations* ~ *Respondeat superior* ~ *Feedback to the board* ~ *Annual budget* ~ *Outside functions* ~ *Planning agencies* ~ *Ex officio member* ~ *Corporate structures* ~ *President of hospital*

INTRODUCTION

At one time, hospital administrators were likely to be chosen from the ranks of the nursing department. In many church-related hospitals, it was common for the administrator to be selected from the ranks of the religious order or from among retired clergymen. These administrators were hardworking and dedicated to patient care, but they were also often trained to follow the physicians' wishes. On the other hand, some administrators, including some of the best qualified the author has known, worked themselves up from the cashier's window through the business office ranks to become the hospital's CEO. It was also common in some hospitals to have a retired businessman or a retired physician assume the CEO position.[1]

Vertical mobility to the administrator rank from other professional levels in the hospital is gone. The first formal educational course for hospital administrators in a university started in the mid-1930s. This occurred as the field of hospital administration became more and more complex following World War II when the demand for trained hospital administrators multiplied. One of the greatest influences on the advancement of the profession of hospital administration was the American College of Hospital Administrators (ACHA), founded in 1933. The college encourages high standards of education and ethics, and only those administrators who meet the College's requirements are admitted as members.[2] Today, formal training of hospital administrators is provided by a number of universities in the United States and Canada. These universities offer graduate degrees in hospital or health care administration.

The training program for hospital administrators covers three general areas: (1) administrative theory, (2) study of certain components of health care services and medical care, and (3) the study of hospital functions, including the organization and management within the hospital and the role of the hospital in the larger picture of health care delivery systems.[3]

FUNCTIONS OF THE ADMINISTRATOR

The main role of the hospital administrator or CEO is to coordinate the facilities of the hospital with its resources so as to allow the medical care mission of the institution to be most efficiently and effectively carried out. Since hospitals are also businesses, their services are capable of being measured by business yardsticks. The administrator's responsibility is to handle and manage the tangibles of money, personnel, and materials. In the view of the ACHA, the responsibility of the governing body or the board of trustees is to function in a judgmental or deliberative fashion. According to the ACHA, "the governing authority appoints a chief executive responsible for the performance of all functions of the institution and accountable to the governing authority. The chief executive, as the head of the organization, is responsible for all functions including a medical staff, nursing division, technical division, and general services division which will be necessary to assure the quality of patient care."[4]

There should be only one person at the head of the hospital. This person usually has the title of administrator, but in some hospitals the CEO may be titled director, president, or executive vice-president.

OUTSIDE AND INSIDE FUNCTIONS

The hospital administrator of the 1930s and 1940s dealt primarily with the internal operations of the hospital. The administrator was concerned with matters that directly affected the patients treated at the hospital. This involved bargaining with employees, developing proper benefit packages, and determining the best methods and techniques to manage the institution. However, in the 1950s and into the 1960s and 1970s, changes occurred in the hospital. Increasingly strong labor unions, third party payers (Blue Cross among them), and governmental agencies all began to impact significantly on the hospital industry. During this period, the role of the administrator became a dual one, dealing with both the inside and outside aspects of hospital management. More sophisticated and specialized management was required to operate a hospital effectively. The CEO became more involved in activities outside the hospital. Today the hospital administration has to strike the proper balance between outside and inside activities.

Inside Activities

Traditionally, it has been the hospital administrator's job to attend to those tasks in the hospital that directly affect the patients' well-being in the hospital. For example, it is the responsibility of the administrator to see that the building and the facilities are in adequate order and that the personnel are qualified to fill their specific job requirements. Legally, the administrator must answer for the acts of employees under the principle of *respondeat superior*.

Another very important and time-consuming aspect of the administrator's job is the relationship with the physicians on the medical staff. One of the crucial tasks of the administrator in this regard is to be an appropriate and effective communicator. The administrator must keep the physicians on the staff informed of the happenings in the hospital and the community that will affect the hospital and the physician's practices. As the agent of the hospital board, the administrator also must intervene in the doctor-patient relationship if there is a violation of law, of medical ethics or morals, or of the hospital rules and regulations.

The administrator has the important function of keeping the governing body informed. After receiving general policies from the governing body, it is the administrator's responsibility to provide proper feedback to the board so that the trustees can be assured that the organization and the functioning of the hospital are in harmony with the mission of the hospital. Frequently, the bane of the administrator's existence is considered to be the job of attending meetings. Yet meetings are important—whether they be with the governing body and its committees, the medical staff, or employees—in order to pass on and communicate ideas, thoughts, policies, and procedures. Additionally, meetings allow the administrator to keep in touch with all constituencies.

A classic responsibility of the hospital administrator is financial. It is the administrator's responsibility to prepare an annual budget for approval by the governing body. The budget must be defended and sold to the hospital board. Pertinent facts about third party reimbursement, rates, and costs must be defined. The financial reports, as well as the budget, must be correlated with the medical care and the quality of that care in the institution. It is the administrator's responsibility, once the budget has been approved, to provide regular and detailed monthly financial reports to the governing body on the status of the hospital; this will include certain financial statements as well as a summary of statistical achievements for the month and the year to date.

Outside Activities

The outside functions of the administrator may be varied and numerous but can be categorized under the following general topics: community activities, governmental relations, social and educational activities, and planning. The administrator is the agent of the board of trustees, who are accountable to the community served by the hospital. The CEO should show leadership, not only within the hospital but outside in the community. This includes a role in educating the community on hospital matters. This can be done in concert with a public relations effort through brochures and pamphlets. It frequently is done through small group conferences or speaking engagements.

With the passage of the Medicare legislation in 1966, the role of government in hospitals has greatly increased. It is the administrator's job to stay on top of changes in governmental funding and planning laws. Frequently, administrators must deal outside the hospital with these funding and planning agencies, whether they be local, state, or federal. If the hospital is involved in a building campaign, the administrator will often have to spend a great deal of time with various state and regional planning agencies and approving bodies (health systems agencies). The responsibility of planning, rehearsing, and discussing the hospital's building plans and future growth plans with outside agencies falls primarily to the administrator. The JCAH and licensing agencies, though they may not be directly related to governmental agencies, can have a major impact on the hospital. It is the administrator's job to maintain close and positive working relationships with these outside reviewing and approving bodies.

Administrators have a responsibility, on behalf of the hospital and the hospital's image, to initiate community health care activities, for example, health fairs and health screening. These activities bring them into contact with the community. As part of their outside role, administrators should try to make contacts with key members in the community. They have an obligation to improve their skills through continuing education. Professional administrators should attend conferences, conventions, educational programs, and courses to strengthen their knowledge of the field and to transfer this knowledge to their hospitals.

KEY RELATIONSHIPS

An administrator must pay close attention to three important relationships: with the medical staff, with the governing body, and with hospital employees.

Relationship with the Medical Staff

For better or for worse, the administrator is a partner with the physicians in delivering health care in the modern hospital. The hospital provides the necessary facilities and personnel to aid the physician in the practice of medicine. The physician—and only the physician—can admit the patients to the hospital. Thus, a necessary partnership is forged.

The best circumstances between the administrator and the medical staff exist when there is a mutual understanding, respect, and trust between the two parties. Each has a separate role in the hospital and can learn from the other. Both parties in their own way are striving to improve the hospital and patient care. Administrators who foster sound relations with the medical staff do so to keep their medical staff informed.

Administrators should keep their staff informed on organizational changes, board policies, and decisions that affect them and their patients. Physicians who understand the reasons for certain policies and decisions will tend to be more supportive. On the other hand, administrators should be sensitive to the medical staff's need for self-governance and support that need. There is a potential for conflicts and tensions between the administrator and the medical staff. Some of these tensions may be natural, since the physicians' interests tend to be directed primarily to the patient and the physicians' own economic survival. The administrators' interests tend to be broader in terms of the entire hospital, their relationships with all the employees, and the financial viability of the institution. These two objectives may in fact not necessarily be in concert.

Members of the medical staff have natural fears; they wonder if the hospital is truly understanding of their problems. Administrators will experience natural frustrations in their relationships with various physicians and their attitudes. These sources of conflict can be varied and many; but the culprit, catalyst, and source of many of the tensions and frustrations that exist might be brought about by poor communications between the administrator and the medical staff. Misunderstandings flourish when effective communication is put in a secondary position. Administrators *must* communicate with their medical staffs—that is a key function of their role. They must be negotiators and integrators in their relationships with the medical staff. Although friction may exist, it is by no means the normal state of affairs in hospital administration and should be minimized. There should be no dividing lines between these two groups; there should be singleness of purpose, enabling the hospital to move ahead in its program much more effectively.

The medical staff views the administrator as a catalyst in management activities, as an implementer, one who is able to provide the physicians' tools in the right place and at the right time to enable them to carry out their work in the hospital. They see the administrator as being accountable for the handling of these resources. This is a valid perception by the medical staff.

Relationship with the Board of Trustees

Boards of trustees give administrators their ultimate authority; boards hire them and can also fire them. The administrator is delegated the authority to administer the affairs of the hospital. Though this relationship is one of employee/employer, in actuality the two parties—the administrator and the board—function as partners. The administrator must turn the board's power into administrative action within the hospital. Just as with the medical staff, communication with the board is critical to the administrator's proper functioning and to the future of the hospital. It is not unheard of to have overzealous, impatient board members cross over into the role of the administrator and start to direct the activities of the hospital themselves. Depending upon the background of the board, this could be a conditioned reflex from the board members' business activities. This can be a difficult problem for the administrator to deal with.

Administrators, on the other hand, have also been known to exceed their authority and to establish policies without the approval of the board. However, both of these circumstances tend to be limited and unique to the field and are not common among hospitals. Indeed, the partnership relationship between the board and the administrator has been solidified through the placement of the CEO as a voting member on many governing boards of hospitals. This is a common occurrence in industry, where the CEO is also a member of the board of directors and is an equal among equals, not just a hired employee. Typically, when administrators are members of boards, they have the title of president under the chairman of the board. CEOs can become active, with voting privileges, or as ex officio members on key board committees, including the nominating, bylaws, and planning committees. However, the CEO should not be the chairman of the board; the trustees on the board are stewards for the community, and the nature of this stewardship should not permit the administrator, an employee of the hospital, to be the chairman.

Relationship with Employees

The employees are the working force of the hospital. Within this group there is a variety of complex human factors, personalities, educational backgrounds, and expertise. The administrator's job is to coordinate this heterogeneous work force into a group with a single mission. Employees regard administrators as their work leaders, and they are expected to fill this role. Administrators have an image to uphold in the hospital; they are perceived as authority figures, as people of action who are supposed to make decisions with speed and wisdom. Employees respond best when they feel they are being brought into the communications link and that they are not being treated arbitrarily. One of the key roles of the administrator is to make the employees aware of the critical nature of their services in the mission of the hospital. This is easier with the nurses and others who deal directly with patients, but the administrator must continually inform all employees of their importance to the whole mission of the hospital. Again, as with the medical staff and the board of trustees, communication is a key to a successful relationship with the employees.

The administrator has the ultimate authority to employ, direct, discipline, and dismiss employees, though this is generally delegated to middle managers and department heads. Because of this, the administrator has a special relationship with department heads. Through the department heads, the administrator executes the rules and regulations concerning the employees' work duties. On the other hand, the administrator has the responsibility to provide the proper organization as well as a safe work environment within the hospital. The administrator must be sensitive to employee needs and see that the personnel are compensated adequately for their effort.

TITLES OF THE ADMINISTRATOR

As can be seen, the modern hospital administrator is not simply the handmaiden of the accounting department of the hospital. In days past, the CEO may have been called the superintendent or director. In recent years, hospitals have been experimenting with new corporate structures for the administrator. In many institutions, the CEO has been given the title of president or executive vice-president rather than administrator because it was felt that the title of administrator did not accurately convey a description of that job's modern role.

Through a combination of tradition and convention in the hospital field, the word *administrator* has come to mean the person in charge. Over recent years, the title has been increasingly replaced by the term *chief executive officer*. The change has come about because the title administrator no longer fits the facts. The title of CEO implies a fully qualified, professionally trained manager. In contrast the title of administrator has come to denote a ministerial role; it has come to be associated with hospital operations. Boards of trustees that continue to refer to the CEO as the administrator are sometimes thought to support the old-fashioned concept of the administrator as the chief bookkeeper and the one who buys equipment for the physicians.

Local variations of the CEO title abound. In some cases, the job includes the role of executive director, executive vice-president, or president of the hospital. It is important to know what is behind the titles of administrator and CEO. In some cases, the title of administrator may be used to describe an individual in charge of hospital operations who reports to the CEO.

NOTES

1. Robert Cunningham, Jr., *Governing Hospitals: Trustees and the New Accountabilities* (Chicago, Ill.: American Hospital Association, 1976), p. 88.

2. Ibid., p. 88.

3. Jonathan Rikich, Beaufort Longest, and Thomas O'Donovan, *Managing Health Care Organizations* (Philadelphia, Pa.: W.B. Saunders Co., 1977), p. 189.

4. American College of Hospital Administrators, *Principles of Appointment and Tenure of Chief Executive Officers* (Chicago, Ill.: American College of Hospital Administrators, 1973).

Part III

Doorways to the Hospital

Chapter 6

Outpatient Areas

Key Terms

Outpatient ≈ Block appointments ≈ Specialty clinics ≈ Referred outpatients ≈ Ambulatory surgery ≈ Medical office building (MOB) ≈ Group practice ≈ Professional corporations (PCs) ≈ JCAH ambulatory standards

INTRODUCTION

There is some disagreement and lack of uniformity as to precisely what is meant by the hospital outpatient area. With the growth of newer concepts in ambulatory medicine, it is especially difficult to define an outpatient area. There is a feeling among some hospital insiders that "hospital outpatient departments have come to be characterized as diffuse, disorganized, busy places pushing and pumping along in their own peculiar cumbersome way physically stuck alongside the 'real in-patient hospital.' "[1] Though there is still confusion as to exactly what fits into the outpatient activities area, some elements are generally understood to belong. Traditional hospital management includes three hospital-related outpatient functions: outpatient clinics, the hospital emergency room, and the special diagnostic and treatment services (laboratory, x-ray, and physical therapy). In addition, there are other types of outpatient medical care delivery, such as ambulatory surgicenters, medical office buildings, and outreach activities (such as store-front clinics and neighborhood health centers).

CLINICS

The history of the hospital outpatient clinic parallels the development of hospitals themselves. In 1752, the Pennsylvania Hospital of Philadelphia opened the first hospital clinic. This was followed by clinics established at the Philadelphia

Dispensary in 1786 and then at other sites through the eighteenth century. These clinics primarily served the urban poor who did not have access to private physicians at that time. Over most of the past 200 years there has been very little change in the nature of the urban hospital clinic. There are, however, wide variations in types of clinics, ranging from an array of very sophisticated, "middle-class," private physician offices to the large urban teaching hospitals manned by house staffs. In the urban areas clinics continue to serve mostly the indigent and to provide a medical resource for those who do not have access to private physicians.

Though there are wide differences in the actual handling of outpatients in hospital clinics, there are some generalizations that can be made about the larger urban clinics. Many of them historically had very modest and spartan atmospheres. Also, their appointment systems were in the main group or block appointment systems. Frequently there were long waiting periods before a patient was seen. Today, much of the care rendered in the larger urban teaching hospitals is given by hospital house staffs, and therefore the continuity of private physician care is lacking. Sometimes the interests of the physicians tend to be more toward teaching and research, and a "guinea pig syndrome" has evolved in some hospitals. Some hospitals have moved toward operating hospital clinics by private physician groups. This has tended to improve the continuity of care, the physical facility, and the social and psychological acceptance of clinic medicine by the patient.

Hospital clinics generally follow the lines of specialization within the hospital medical staff. This means that hospitals offer outpatient clinics in medicine, surgery, obstetrics, gynecology, and pediatrics in addition to the basic services. In the more technologically advanced and esoteric teaching centers, there can be as many as 50 or 60 different specialty clinics meeting some time during each month.

Over the last several years, hospitals have removed "hard wooden benches" and have made an effort to modernize their facilities. Individual appointment systems are replacing the block systems, and family practice clinics and other primary care clinics have added to continuity of care. The number of patients is being pared down, with new patients receiving considerably more time for their initial visit.

Due primarily to the great increase in emergency department visits and associated nonhospital clinic ambulatory visits, the hospital's supporting services—such as laboratory, x-ray, and physical therapy—have provided a major source of support for the hospital's outpatients. This whole area has been growing. Traditionally, when patients were referred for laboratory or x-ray studies or for physical therapy treatments, rather than being registered as clinic patients, the hospital recorded these patients as "referred outpatients." The work referred to the ancillary services supporting the outpatient activity and the clinic patients referred to these ancillary services have been on the rise; this is a significant factor in a hospital's revenue picture. One study showed outpatient activity in the various ancillary service departments as follows: laboratory, 17 percent; diagnostic radiology, 47 percent; therapeutic radiology, 89 percent; nuclear medicine, 29 percent; and physical therapy, 37 percent.[2]

Because of the deficit financial nature of hospital clinics and the emergency departments, hospital controllers and hospital administrators frequently seek to have third party payers pick up their proper portion of the bills for the medical indigent outpatients or to hasten dissolution of their clinics through establishment of private group practices or the sharing of services.

AMBULATORY SURGERY

Hospital and consumers (that is, HSAs) alike are looking for the optimal way to deliver health care. Ambulatory surgery (outpatient surgery) over the last decade has shown increased usage and a great promise in hospitals. Ambulatory surgery is defined as surgery (generally of a minor nature) that does not require the patient to remain overnight in the hospital. The ambulatory surgery might be performed totally in the hospital's operating room; it could also be performed in a special surgical clinic or in a short-term unit (short procedure unit). Though we tend to believe that ambulatory surgery is a new type of delivery of care, Thomas O'Donovan, in his description of ambulatory surgery in *Ambulatory Surgical Centers, Development and Management,* points out that a Dr. Nichol in 1909 described to the British Medical Association several thousand operations performed on ambulatory patients in a Scottish hospital.[3] However, it was not until the 1960s, as hospitals, physicians, and third party payers began critically to review the matter, that many other factors came to bear on the issue of ambulatory surgery.

The provision of outpatient or ambulatory surgical facilities for patients offers numerous advantages to the hospital:

1. It allows the institution to shift patients from highly occupied inpatient beds, which better utilizes hospital resources;
2. It frees costly inpatient beds for the more acutely ill that otherwise might be occupied by short-term surgical patients; this also permits the more expensive inpatient facilities to be more effectively utilized;
3. It provides the hospital with the ability to staff more flexibly, especially if the short-term unit or ambulatory center is near the Emergency Room;
4. It permits maximum utilization of personnel and resources in the Operating Room;
5. The ambulatory surgery precludes one day admissions from staying overnight, thereby reducing the operating expenses which would be assigned to the round-the-clock staffing of that patient;

6. By ambulatory surgical patients being scheduled it allows the nursing staff and Operating Room staff to tailor their resources to predictable needs;
7. Frequently ambulatory surgery centers use abbreviated medical records and billing forms thereby reducing paper work and clerical processing time;
8. The ambulatory surgery, by reducing the inpatient beds, lowers future capital construction costs for hospital facilities.[4]

In addition to providing advantages to the institution, ambulatory surgery saves patients valuable time away from work. In many cases it reduces the inpatient stay of two or three days to six or eight hours. In very crowded circumstances, moreover, patients who might have to wait on a hospital admission list for elective surgery can have minor surgery performed through the ambulatory surgery center, thereby reducing the time for surgery. Not having to stay overnight is an important advantage for patients who are parents with children, since the parent and the child may both be apprehensive about sleeping in the hospital. With less time spent in the hospital, charges to patients are less than they would be for a 24-hour or 48-hour hospital stay.[5]

MEDICAL OFFICE BUILDINGS

With the changing patterns of ambulatory medicine, physicians as well as hospital management have had to rethink the conventional ways of rendering service and providing resources. In many communities the traditional office with one physician and one nurse has been rapidly disappearing. Physicians have learned that banding together in medical office buildings, sharing overhead and, in some instances, staff and other resources such as laboratory and x-ray, has provided an efficient and economical way to practice outpatient medicine.[6]

Hospitals also have recognized that efficient outpatient care can be rendered in a systemized, well-planned medical office building. The medical office building is usually a separate building, but it could include segments of existing hospitals, such as floors, wings, or towers that have been made into medical office building suites. Medical office building concepts provide an interesting example of a winning situation where the innovation is good for the hospital, the physician, and the patient.

Why should a hospital be involved in a medical office building? One of the reasons is that it stabilizes the office location of key staff physicians who might shift their offices or their allegiance to other hospitals or other communities. Also, it gives the hospital an additional tool for physician recruitment. The presence of a viable medical office building on the hospital campus or within the hospital has been shown to increase the patient census at the hospital. Frequently, hospitals find disincentives in the fact that a neighboring, competing hospital has a building and they do not. In such cases, hospitals find themselves competing just to keep up with other competing hospitals.[7]

The actual organization, financial structure, and legal structure for medical office building complexes vary. There are essentially four models: (1) The hospital owns and maintains the facility. (2) The medical office building is owned by the physicians, and the hospital acts as a partner to secure loans and financing arrangements. (3) The physicians and an outside developer own the building and lease the land from the hospital. (4) The physicians and an outside developer own the building, and the hospital leases space from the physician-developer group. Though these four models are available, recent studies show that over 80 percent of the medical office buildings under construction are being built by hospitals.[8]

The financing of a medical office building will undoubtedly cost several millions of dollars. It could create a real fiscal concern for hospitals and hospital board members. A hospital planner might also be involved, since the development could involve a certificate-of-need application with planning agencies. It is important for managers, board members, and planners to remember that generally the medical office building will increase the hospital's x-ray, laboratory, and other ancillary revenues as well as generally increase inpatient occupancy. This will result in potentially greater operating surpluses for the hospital and an improved cash flow. Frequently, the interior space of medical office buildings is the responsibility of the individual physicians or physician groups, since having the physician owners make lease-hold improvements offers them tax advantages.

The concept of a medical office building associated with a hospital is an idea whose time has come. The concept allows for patient care on an ambulatory basis to be a partnership between hospitals as providers and physicians as providers. In these circumstances, the patient frequently receives a one-stop service under the umbrella of quality care supported by the medical staff in the hospital. Viable medical office buildings permit physician groups to establish an excellent nucleus for the development of health maintenance organizations.

GROUP PRACTICE

Medical group practice is defined as "the application of medical services by three or more physicians formally organized to provide medical care, consultation, diagnosis and/or treatment through the joint use of equipment and personnel and with the income from medical practice distributed in accordance with methods previously determined by members of the group. Groups are usually organized as single owner groups, partnerships, professional corporations (PC's), associations or foundations."[9] There are subdefinitions of medical groups—such as single specialty groups, general practice groups, and groups made up of various specialties. Group practices have had a significant impact on hospitals that deliver outpatient services. It has been noted that, "As recently as four years ago, physician groups provided some aspect of outpatient services in a little more than a third of the United States community hospitals."[10] Two of the more recent and largest growing specialty groups are the emergency department groups that render services to a hospital's emergency rooms and primary care service groups that are based either in the hospital itself or in the hospital's medical office building complex.

The concept of group practice in medicine began to evolve around the turn of the century. Prior to that time, physicians joined together to practice medicine, but they did not consider themselves as an organized group practice. C. Rufus Rodium provided a great deal of insight into the evolution of group practice when he noted:

> Specialization in knowledge and skill in the use of capital investment in medical practice are causes and not results of group practice. The scientific and economic aspects of present day health service make it necessary that the various phases of diagnosis and treatment be coordinated. The general hospital is a natural site for the greatest development of group practice in America. The medical specialists are already spending a great deal of time in hospitals in the care of patients who need bed care during a portion of their diagnosis and treatment. The hospitals contain the greatest portion of specialized equipment for diagnosis and treatment, together with a full-time staff trained to use the facilities under medical supervision.[11]

The American Medical Association (AMA) estimates that 23 percent of physicians in the United States, excluding house staff, are engaged in group practice. The AMA indicates that approximately 18 percent are in free-standing medical groups, 2 percent in prepaid groups, and 12 percent in hospital-based group practices.[12]

Some of the reasons physicians join a group practice are the ease of consultation; the reduction of administrative overhead and duties by hiring trained clerical personnel; the opportunities for physicians to recruit newer physicians to their group; financial security and financial incentives for the physicians; less use of hospital facilities by the physicians; improved clinical results, especially in prenatal mortality; and the tendency to improve professional competency. Some of the criticisms offered are increased overutilization of the outpatient facilities; the reduction of personnel; less personal relationships between the physician and the patient; a too highly structured organization to really benefit the physician; the gearing of services toward the acute and categorical illnesses rather than individual patient care; and case loads that tend to be mostly paying patients, that is, a reduction in the rendering of free care.[13]

STANDARDS OF ACCREDITATION

The JCAH has two different and separate sets of standards for evaluating ambulatory health care. One set applies to hospital-sponsored outpatient service programs; the other applies to free-standing ambulatory care programs. This says something about the future of outpatient medicine, in that the hospital and the private sector (particularly private physicians) each has its own definite needs and the JCAH has recognized this with two independent sets of criteria for evaluating quality. In 1976, the JCAH accepted essentially the quality standards for free-standing groups that had already been promulgated by the American Group Practice Association.

At first the JCAH standards, published in 1973, applied only to hospital outpatient departments. These standards were separate and distinct from the standards of the JCAH that applied to emergency departments. However it is optional for a hospital to have an outpatient service, and a hospital may still qualify for JCAH standards in the absence of an outpatient service. The outpatient standards are integrated with the JCAH standards used for other functional areas of the hospital.

The JCAH 1978 standards for free-standing ambulatory services are geared to apply to outpatient activities irrespective of their organizational sponsorship. The standards were expanded from their initial concentration on group medical matters to include a wide spectrum of ambulatory facilities, including ambulatory surgical facilities, health maintenance organizations, community health centers, and other similar patient care services.

NOTES

1. Richard A. Berman and Thomas W. Mohoney, "Where Does Real Fiscal Control of the Outpatient Department Lie? " *Hospitals, J.A.H.A.,* March 16, 1977, p. 99.
2. "Study Shows That Outpatient Department Is Major Source of Hospital Revenue," *Hospitals, J.A.H.A.,* November, 1979, p. 46.
3. Thomas R. O'Donovan, ed., *Ambulatory Surgical Centers* (Germantown, Md.: Aspen Systems Corp., 1976). p. 4.
4. I. Donald Snook, Jr., "A Short Term Care-Unit Bridge the Gap Between Inpatient/Outpatient Facilities," *Hospital Financial Management,* March 1973, p. 26.
5. Ibid., p. 26.
6. O'Donovan, *Ambulatory Surgical Centers,* pp. 14-17.
7. "Ambulatory Surgical Facility" (Hollywood, Fla.)
8. Marion S. Kessler and Susan Ashby, "Hospital Landlords: Trends in Leasing Medical Office Space," *The Hospital Medical Staff,* July 1979, p. 30.
9. U.S. Department of Health, Education, and Welfare, "Medical Group Practices," *Health Resources Statistics, 1972-73, HEW Publication 73-1509,* 1973, p. 485.

10. "Acceptance of Hospital-Related Group Practices Vary Widely," *Hospitals, J.A.H.A.*, May 1, 1979, p. 53.
11. Committee on Medical Care Teaching of the Association of Teachers of Preventive Medicine, ed., *Readings in Medical Care* (Chapel Hill, N.C.: University of North Carolina Press, 1958), p. 322.
12. Gregg W. Downey, "Group Practice: Profits and Perils," *Modern Health Care,* January 1979, p. 16m.
13. James W. Manier, "Group Practice: A Mechanism for Health Care Delivery in the 1970's," *The Internist,* May 1970, p. 20.

Chapter 7

The Emergency Department

Key Terms

Accident room ~ *Emergency Department committee* ~ *Compulsory rotation* ~
Rotating panel ~ *Pontiac Plan* ~ *Alexandria Plan* ~ *Categorization* ~
Emergency Department log ~ *Wilmington General Hospital v. Manlow* ~ *Disaster plan* ~ *Free-standing emergency room*

INTRODUCTION

In the early days of hospitals, an "accident room" was a necessity in the medical institution. The accident room was the place to treat patients who were truly injured with surgical problems, automobile accidents, home accidents, or accidents on the job. At that time, hospital management viewed the accident room as a necessary evil to provide the service necessary for the community. The general practitioners, surgeons, obstetricians, and pediatricians had very little use for the concept of accident rooms. Such rooms were generally staffed by the hospital intern, who was possibly the most inexperienced person to deal with accident situations. Typically, there were registered nurses to support the intern. A recent medical journal described the accident room this way: "It was born in the basement and was relegated to the basement until the late 1960's."[1]

Things started to change after World War II. As medical schools and teaching hospitals began to produce superspecialties and the general practitioner began to shrink from the medical scene, it was not long before patients discovered that they had nowhere to turn for the usual minor complaints and illnesses. The path of least resistance and the one frequently open was the hospital accident room. The accident room became a walk-in medical clinic in many communities.

The emergency room has a split personality. It can handle acute trauma, and it also is available for walk-in medical patients. The ideal emergency department is one that specializes in trauma care. It is open 24 hours a day and is well staffed by competent, experienced physicians and nurses. A background in trauma training has to be complemented by training in internal medicine, cardiology, and possibly psychiatry. Presently emergency rooms throughout the country are facing a crisis. Since World War II there has been a continual increase in emergency room visits, making effective emergency department management more difficult. For the last ten years, emergency room visits have increased 175 percent, yet studies show that as high as 60 percent of these visits represent nonemergencies.[2]

THE BOOM IN PATIENT VOLUME

The annual number of patients visiting a hospital emergency room in the United States is reported to be three times that of a decade ago. One reason for the increase is a shortage of physicians. Over the last 15 years, the number of general practitioners in private practice has dwindled from 95,000 to 68,000, of whom only 45,000 are now treating patients full time. Reviewers have indicated that people of the western world are depending more upon the emergency room than physician medical care. Americans have become more migratory, moving from city to city so frequently that they have little opportunity to establish rapport with an individual physician. It has been noted that "the public has come to look upon the Emergency Department as the community medical center where anyone may come with any complaint at any hour of the day or night and expect prompt and courteous attention as his due."[3] A study conducted by the Lober organization indicates that "two-thirds of the American public regard the hospital emergency department as being interchangeable with a physician's office for general treatment capabilities."[4] The survey found that the main reason many people prefer the hospital emergency room for treatment is that they think hospitals have better treatment facilities than physicians' offices.[5] Emergency rooms are being used as afterhours' physicians' offices and have become 24-hour outpatient clinics. This places a heavy burden on the facilities, space, staff, and finances of the hospital.

On average, emergency room visits show a five to six percent increase each year. In 1972, there were 60.1 million visits; in 1978, the number was 82.8 million. Traditionally, the hospital has been geared to provide inpatient care, but with the increased demands for emergency and other ambulatory care services, management has had to find ways to integrate the demand for these growing programs into the hospital's future. The emergency room's skyrocketing volume is placing pressure on hospital planners to find appropriate ambulatory care settings to serve their communities. One reason the increased volume is placing pressure on the hospital is that a significant number of the hospital's inpatients are admitted through the emergency room. Some hospitals report as many as one-third of their total admissions come from the emergency room. A hospital's size, location of emergency department, staffing arrangements, and ownership affect the number of inpatients coming from the emergency department.

WHAT BRINGS PATIENTS TO THE EMERGENCY ROOM?

As physicians have turned to formal appointment types of practices, emergency rooms have become the place for informal walk-in treatment. A Blue Cross survey in Michigan showed 23 percent of the patients who visited the emergency room came directly to the hospital without calling a physician because they did not believe a physician would be available. Another 12 percent went to the emergency room after they were unable to reach their private physician.

The greatest concentration of medical facilities in any community is found in the hospital. To assure immediate and adequate care, modern physicians prefer to render service where they have access to these resources. The same Michigan survey showed that 23 percent of all patients were treated by their own physician in the emergency room. Nearly 19 percent of the patients were instructed by their physicians to meet them at the hospital.

For a mobile population like that of the United States, the use of emergency services for family care has become a way of life. The relocation of families from one area to another has had a profound impact on the use of emergency rooms. When an illness strikes before the family has had time to select a private physician, the hospital becomes the natural place to seek care.

The move of middle-income families and their physicians to suburban areas has left urban hospitals surrounded by economically disadvantaged families who depend on the hospital for medical care. Still, patients who are financially able to pay for care sometimes choose emergency room services if they live a great distance from a physician's office. Many patients have learned that their medical needs are obtained much more quickly in hospital emergency rooms. A study of families bringing children to the Emergency Pediatric Clinic at Freedman's Hospital in Washington, D.C., showed that the majority were seeking routine medical care. Most of the families lived near the hospital, and most of them did not have private physicians.[6]

ORGANIZATION

The emergency room is generally considered to be an outpatient nursing unit in the hospital organization. However, unlike other hospital nursing units, the medical staff plays a major onsite role in the emergency department and thereby complicates the organization of the emergency room. Typically, the nursing service staffs the emergency room with nursing and auxiliary personnel as they do any other nursing unit. However, since physician coverage is required in the unit (and more recently emergency departments are becoming managed by an emergency department specialist or group), there is a management partnership between physicians and nurses in this unit.

The current organizational trend in emergency rooms is for the unit to be a separate and distinct department under the direction of a full-time physician director. This evolution from a nursing unit within a nursing service to a physician-directed department is more prominent in the larger hospitals that employ full-time physicians to staff the activity. The physicians generally report directly to the medical staff, to the management of the hospital, or through a committee called the emergency department committee of the medical staff. Unlike the inpatient nursing unit, the emergency department committee is frequently a committee of the medical staff that has the task to evaluate and plan the operations of the emergency department by enlisting the opinions and skills of a variety of concerned persons in the hospital. Typically, the emergency department committee is made up of representatives from the medical staff, nursing staff, and administration. This committee formulates the medical-administrative policies to guide the emergency room operations. It also examines the level and quality of emergency care rendered in the department. More recently, under the PSRO medical care evaluation studies requirement, this committee may be involved in analyzing the flow of patients and the relationship of the emergency department patients to the ancillary services, such as x-ray and laboratory.

With the increased number of emergency visits, the trend has been for full-time emergency room physicians to staff the unit. The simplest model for full-time physicians is one in which the hospital pays one or more physicians a flat salary for attending patients. As a rule, the salaried emergency room physician is a hospital employee. Under these circumstances the hospital bills patients for the use of the emergency room as well as for the physician's services.

ADMISSIONS

It is important to realize that the emergency department has a significant impact on the hospital's inpatient population. A study by the American Hospital Association indicates that between 16 and 30 percent of the hospital's admissions come through the emergency department.[7] It has been noted that "not only do emergency admission patients generally remain in the hospital for a longer period of time, but also their admissions usually entail greater use of ancillary services than that which occurs with scheduled patients. Therefore, reliable gauges of the extent to which the emergency department activity is converted to inpatient hospital use are particularly important to planners, administrators, and fiscal intermediaries."[8]

Emergency department patients will follow one of five avenues after coming for service: The patient may (1) be treated and sent home; (2) be treated, held over in the emergency department for observation in the "holding rooms," and then sent home; (3) require emergency surgery, go directly to the operating room, and then to an inpatient unit; (4) be admitted directly to the inpatient unit; or (5) be stabilized in the emergency department and transferred to another hospital for admission.[9]

It is incumbent upon the hospital's medical staff to provide backup support for emergency patients. This is particularly important for patients requiring admission. Under ideal circumstances, medical coverage should be provided by those interested physicians, but hospital circumstances vary and at times it is necessary for the chief of service (medicine or surgery) to establish a mandatory, rotating coverage schedule. In this case, when patients need admission, the physician on the on-call list is notified to offer the patient any specialty care required or to act as the admitting physician for patients who require hospitalization.

PHYSICIAN STAFFING OF THE EMERGENCY ROOM

There are a variety of methods employed to provide physician coverage for hospital emergency rooms. In a very complete article on the topic, James Lifton points out that there are six basic plans with two variations that hospitals can use:

1. Compulsory rotation of the hospital's attending staff. This is the classic method of emergency room physician staffing in hospitals. Under this arrangement, physicians on the medical staff are required to provide coverage on a rotating basis.
2. Voluntary rotation of the attending staff. This is similar to compulsory rotation except not all staff members participate. Only those who volunteer are in the rotation.
3. A rotating panel. This method is used when many physicians request to provide coverage under the voluntary arrangement. The staff is divided into two or more groups or panels which then rotate. Rotating panels are also used in specialty referrals from the emergency department, for example, a panel of general surgeons or internists.
4. House staff coverage. As a teaching device and as a convenience for attending staff physicians, residents and medical students frequently staff the emergency department in large teaching hospitals.
5. A general group contractual plan. This plan originated in Pontiac, Michigan, and is sometimes referred to as the Pontiac Plan. A (relatively) large group of private practitioners contractually agrees

to staff the emergency department while still retaining their individual practices.

6. A specialist group contractual plan. This has been used in Alexandria, Virginia, and is referred to as the Alexandria Plan. This arrangement calls for a (relatively) small group of specialty physicians to staff the emergency department under contract. These physicians do not maintain a private practice.
7. Any combination of the Pontiac and Alexandria Plans.
8. Full-time salaried physicians employed by the hospital. This is a rather common arrangement that does not depend on the size of the hospital or emergency department. Generally, the employed physician does not have a private practice.[10]

It falls to the hospital management and the medical staff to determine the best staffing situation for a hospital. General legislation, shifts in population growth, and additional emphasis on ambulatory medicine are some of the factors to be considered when selecting the proper staffing method.

CATEGORIZATION OF EMERGENCY FACILITIES

Not all hospitals operate emergency rooms, nor are hospitals required to do so by law, regulation, or the JCAH. However, if a hospital does operate an emergency service, it is held to all appropriate rules and regulations of third party agencies. In the early 1970s, various organizations, regions, and states began to review the concept of categorizing the (different) emergency rooms into the levels of care that they are capable of providing. Studies were carried out in the city of Philadelphia and in the northwestern region of Ohio. The National Research Council and the National Academy of Sciences identified four categories of emergency care. Basically the categorization is keyed to the levels and depths of services that each hospital is able to provide, with Type I being the highest level and Type IV the minimal level. Type I major emergency facilities include 24-hour specialists in the hospital in addition to other 24-hour backup services. Type II is the basic emergency facility where the emergency room physician is located in the hospital with certain specialists on call. Type III is the hospital that provides standby emergency facilities with perhaps an emergency-room registered nurse and a physician on call. Type IV is a referral emergency room facility that has only an emergency nurse or medical technician in the hospital and that transfers patients to other facilities for life support systems.[11] The JCAH has outlined the requirements of each type's care level needed for accreditation.

FINANCIAL IMPLICATIONS

Because the emergency room is generally open 24 hours a day, with heavy costs in the area of physician salaries and around-the-clock nursing staff, the hospital must look at the broader implications of having an emergency service. A traditional view of the emergency room is that it is a drain on the economics of the hospital. Depending on the financial status of the outpatients visiting the emergency room, especially in the urban areas, it could be a financial drain. In an average hospital, a significant portion of the inpatients come through the emergency department. In addition, studies have shown that emergency department patients utilize the ancillary services of the hospital. The high use of the ancillary services by both outpatients and inpatients contributes to the increased charge structure and hopefully an improved cash flow for the hospitals.

Typically, one-third of the bill for a hospital emergency department patient stems from the emergency department; the remaining charges are generated through the utilization of the ancillary services.[12] With the use of ancillary services and the element of free care in the outpatient aspect of the emergency rooms, the financial dimension of the emergency department is complex.

It is common for urban emergency rooms to run a high level of bad debts and free care. The principal factor causing this financial drain is the emergency room's third party demographics. Because of the physician availability problem in our urban areas, a large number of welfare (Medicaid) and indigent patients use the emergency room as a substitute primary care physician. In many states, the government's Medicaid outpatient reimbursement formulas do not meet the hospital's costs, thereby leaving the emergency room with a large financial deficit and inadequate cash flow.

The typical patient's bill for a visit to the emergency department may include three different types of charges. First, there is a basic charge that will vary between hospitals; this is the part of the bill that helps pay for the fixed and overhead charges in the department. Second, there may be a separate charge for physicians' services. If the hospital employs the emergency department physician or the house staff is used, there will not be a separate charge for professional services. Third, there may be an ancillary or special services charge for drugs, x-rays, and laboratory work performed.

The emergency room must be viewed in the sense of total hospital impact rather than as a restricted departmental outpatient center. Emergency departments may increase the hospital's census and cash flow in the inpatient area. Improved physical facilities, competent professional staffing, and the image of high quality patient care in the community all seem to add up to increased volume in the hospital's emergency rooms, which then tends to lower the cost per visit.

RECORDS

Good medical and administrative practice demands that the hospital initiate medical records on each patient visiting the emergency room department. It is also necessary for the hospital to protect itself legally. Most emergency department medical records are simplified compared to the extensive inpatient records. Generally, they carry administrative and basic statistical data about the patient with a place for appropriate baseline clinical data, such as blood pressure and temperature, plus a space for physicians' and nurses' notes. Generally the emergency room record is limited to one sheet. If a patient is admitted to the hospital, the emergency room record accompanies the patient and is made a part of the patient's inpatient medical chart. If the patient is not admitted, the emergency room record is retained in the emergency department, and another copy is sent to the medical records department for proper storage. It is common practice in many emergency rooms to have several carbon copies of the medical record. One of the copies is forwarded to the patient's attending physician by the emergency personnel as a professional courtesy and to aid in the patient's future care and continuity of care.

It is typical for emergency departments to maintain a register or log of patients. This is usually an appointment book or a sheet of paper containing such information as the patient's name, date of admission to the emergency room, age, sex, type of medical or surgical problem, and the disposition of the case. The emergency room log provides information for emergency department studies, such as frequency of visits, the nature of the visits, and so forth. When patients arrive at the emergency department with a previous inpatient admission history at that hospital, the physicians and nurses treating the patient will usually request the patient's prior inpatient medical record so that proper treatment can be given to the patient.

LEGAL IMPLICATIONS

Perhaps the most common legal question arising in the emergency department is the issue of treating minors who come to the emergency room without their parents or guardian. Hospitals have to weigh the threat of assault and battery versus the matter of rendering necessary emergency care. Kucera reports the following case:

> In the landmark case of Wilmington General Hospital vs. Manlow, the emergency department nurse refused to admit a four-month-old infant who was seriously ill with diarrhea. His temperature was 102 degrees. The nurse refused to admit the infant because the child's parents did not have an authorization slip from their family physician who had prescribed the medication for the child. The parents took the child home

where he died later that afternoon. The Delaware Supreme Court held
liability on the part of the hospital may be predicated on the refusal of
service to the patient in the case of an unmistakable emergency if the
patient relied upon a well established custom of the hospital to render aid
in such a case.[13]

Following this landmark court decision, many states now maintain that the
hospital holds itself out to the public as a provider of emergency medical services
and that the hospital is accordingly under an obligation to provide emergency care
to any individual who comes for it. Lawyers advise emergency department
physicians that if it is a threat to life and limb it is far better to treat the child even in
the absence of securing parental consent than to send the minor out of the
emergency department.

Another important issue in the area of the hospital liability is the matter of the
hospital's responsibility to inform the emergency department patient clearly in
language that the patient can understand about the type and timing of any recommended followup medical care. Many hospitals, in attempting to adopt this
principle, give the patient written followup instructions to reduce their liability and
to improve communications.

Among some of the other trials and tribulations that arise in the emergency room
is the handling of the angry and combative patient. The angry, uncooperative
patient may want to sign out against medical advice. This could cause a problem
for both the patient and the hospital if the patient needs emergency treatment. One
way to approach this situation is through communication. The staff has to see that
the patient has been injured or ill and must understand the patient's feelings and
accept them. The patient's anger may stem from a brusque physician's commands
or may be a simple reaction to pain.

The first level of handling this problem is through dialogue. Sometimes the aid
of a psychiatrist or the use of medication is necessary. In extreme cases, communication and psychiatric treatment may have to be complemented with the presence
of the police to control the patient. Once the threat to the patient's life or limb is
past, the angry, hostile patient becomes more of a social problem than a medical
problem and should be handled accordingly.

The presence of intoxicated patients in the emergency room usually creates a
sense of turmoil. Such patients can be loud, hostile, demanding, and in general
difficult to deal with. Many times these patients may be escorted into the emergency room by police, often from the scene of a recent accident. Frequently the
police authorities ask for a blood alcohol test. This is a clinical laboratory
procedure to determine the level of alcohol present in the patient's blood at any
given time, the results of which could prove whether the patient was legally
intoxicated. Hospitals must be cautious in permitting blood alcohol tests to be

taken without the patient's concurrence (the patient's signed permission). Since requests for these tests may occur frequently, the emergency room staff must be thoroughly familiar with the local laws, statutes, and regulations that apply to the taking of blood alcohols.

PHYSICAL FACILITIES

It is advisable that the emergency department be located on the ground floor with easy access for patients and ambulances. Generally, it is best to have it separated from the main entrance of the hospital. The emergency department should make its entrance easily visible from the street, for example, with proper lighting and signs. It is very important that the ambulance entrance to the emergency department be large enough to admit one or more ambulances negotiating with stretchers. Emergency rooms should have waiting rooms sufficient for patients and their families and friends as well as telephone areas and rest rooms close by. X-ray and laboratory services should be easily accessible to the emergency department. Over 40 percent of emergency patients require x-rays, and over 20 percent need laboratory studies. If emergency rooms handle a patient volume in excess of 1,000 patients per month or handle an unusually high number of fracture cases, they may have their own x-ray facilities. A portable x-ray apparatus is seldom satisfactory. If an x-ray unit is located within the emergency room, provision must be made for the consultation services of radiology technicians and radiologists.

Generally, the emergency department has at least two or three functional areas. Typically, there is the trauma area where the severely injured surgical cases are handled. There should be a medical examining area nearby and a casting area for orthopedic problems. There should be observation beds for patients who need to stay in the emergency room area (for neurological and other medical reasons). These observation beds can be used as a staying area before the patient moves to the inpatient nursing unit.

It is common for police, ambulance attendants, and at times members of the press to congregate in the emergency room. It is important that these groups be kept away from the clinical work areas. Emergency rooms that are large enough and properly designed will have a small room set aside for these groups that is equipped with a desk, telephone, and chairs. The provision of coffee for them is a welcome addition. Such accommodations promote good public relations. The Committee on Trauma of the American College of Surgeons has published a model of a hospital emergency department that outlines in clear, understandable detail the proper physical facilities requirements and suggests layouts for the emergency department.[14]

HANDLING DISASTERS

It is necessary for hospitals to have a written document that outlines procedures to be followed by hospital staff in the event of a community catastrophe or disaster, such as a train wreck, airplane crash, large industrial accident, major fire, or natural disasters. The JCAH requires each hospital to have a written disaster plan and to rehearse the plan at least twice annually.

Hospitals should be prepared for three kinds of disasters. The first is an internal hospital disaster, such as an explosion or major fire. The second is an external disaster, such as a hurricane, tornado, flood, or transportation accident. The third is a forewarned disaster, such as the receipt of a large number of patients from a neighboring hospital that has had to evacuate.

Key areas in a disaster plan include the reception area and the triage area, usually near the emergency department. Triage comes from the French word meaning to sort out. It is common for emergency departments to sort out (screen) patients upon their arrival. They may be sorted out to a walk-in clinic or a trauma treatment area, or be admitted directly to the hospital. There also must be a room for families and the press. There must be a plan for the evacuation of patients who are able to leave and give up their beds for more seriously ill patients. There should be a temporary morgue if it is not already located in the hospital's present morgue. There must be an understanding of how communications will flow during the disaster. In addition, a labor pool with assignments for physicians should be ready to set in motion. External traffic control and police protection must be considered. Finally, places to secure additional medical supplies and food for the duration must be known.

THE FUTURE

The trend of an increase in emergency department visits will undoubtedly continue because the needs of the people who come to the emergency room have not been addressed as yet. Patients will continue to be approximately 80 percent nonemergency with the remaining cases emergency; only 5 percent of the total will be in critical need of care. Some hospitals have opened satellite emergency departments, especially in rural areas where it is difficult to recruit general practitioners and hospital resources are not readily available.

The proprietary medical sector has become involved in ambulatory surgery centers. Some years ago, Dr. Robert Gordon opened the first free-standing proprietary emergency room near Providence, Rhode Island. He experienced some difficulty among the established medical community and some of the town fathers, but the Warwick Emergency Department has been seeing high volumes of patients. Generally, free-standing emergency rooms are able to offer their services at less cost than hospital emergency departments. The bulk of the patients in both satellite and free-standing emergency rooms are there for treatment of minor ailments, for example, a foreign body in the eye or a laceration requiring a few stitches. These facilities also provide care for patients whose doctor is out of town or otherwise unavailable. They do not encourage treatment for patients suffering from cardiac arrest or other life-threatening conditions. Such patients should be brought directly to a hospital emergency room. It appears that free-standing emergency rooms will continue to grow at a steady rate.

Finally, the future of emergency services will dictate some categorization. In fact, the state of Illinois Hospital Licensing Act now requires three types of emergency treatment services: (1) comprehensive; (2) basic emergency service, where at least one physician is in the emergency room at all times; and (3) a standby emergency service, where at least a registered nurse is on duty and patients can be transferred in life-threatening circumstances.

NOTES

1. Eugene J. Riley, "Emergency Evolution," *St. Joseph's Hospital Bulletin,* 1977.
2. *American Medical Association News,* September 8, 1966.
3. Roy Hudenburg, *Planning the Community Hospital* (New York, N.Y.: McGraw-Hill Book Co., 1967).
4. American Hospital Association, "Hospital Week," April 15, 1977.
5. Ibid.
6. "Emergency Crisis—Why Case Loads Are Up," *Medical World News* 6 (1965): 64.
7. Henry J. Smith, "Utilization of Podiatric Emergency Services of Freedman's Hospital for Routine Medical Care," *Journal of the National Medical Association* 58 (1966): 143-5.
8. Marion S. Kessler and Karen C. Wilson, "Emergency Department Key Factor in Hospital Admissions," *Hospitals, JAHA,* December 16, 1978, p. 87.
9. Ibid.
10. James G. Lifton, "Eight Ways to Provide Physician Coverage of the Emergency Room and How to Tell Which Is Best," *Modern Hospital,* October 1973, pp. 79-82.
11. Maurice A. Schnieker, "Categorization of Hospital Emergency Departments—How It Was Done in Ohio," *Philadelphia Medicine,* March 20, 1973, p. 210.
12. Karl G. Mangold, "The Financial Realities of EMS," *Hospitals, JAHA,* May 1973, p. 92.
13. William R. Kucera, "Narrow Definition of Emergency Can Spell Litigation," *The Hospital Medical Staff,* September 1978, p. 23.
14. The Committee on Trauma of the American College of Surgeons, *A Model of a Hospital Emergency Department* (Chicago, Ill.: American College of Surgeons), August 1967.

Chapter 8

The Admitting Department

Key Terms

Patient information booklets ∼ Patient's bill of rights ∼ Emergency admissions ∼ Urgent admissions ∼ Elective admissions ∼ Public Law 92-603 (PSRO Legislation) ∼ Admitting criteria ∼ Preadmission ∼ Preadmission testing ∼ Informed consent ∼ Bed allocation policy

INTRODUCTION

The admitting department has changed over the last decade. It once was a relatively easy matter for the patient or the patient's family to give the admissions' clerk the routine factual information necessary to admit the patient. Those days are gone. A host of external factors—including the legal system, the third party payer, governmental control, and review programs—have changed the role and the task of the admissions officer.

THE DEPARTMENT'S ROLE IN PUBLIC RELATIONS

The movement toward patients' rights and the recognition of the hospital as a very competitive business have made the admissions office a key public relations arm of the hospital. Public relations are involved at all points of entry to the hospital—the admissions office, the emergency department, the hospital's clinics, and the private doctor's office in the medical office building of the hospital. Patients should find at all points of entry staff who are at all times sympathetic, understanding, courteous, and professional. This is important to maintain and improve the hospital's image.

A patient's impression of the hospital begins at the admitting office. A positive image can be generated through patient information booklets or brochures that are either distributed before or at the admission of the patient; frequently these are given to the patient's family and to visitors as well. A booklet for patients outlining the "do's" and "don'ts" of the hospital stay will make the patient's hospitalization a bit more comfortable and will help alleviate anxiety. Several years ago the American Hospital Association developed a "Patient's Bill of Rights" that explained a hospital's obligations to patients and clarified the relationships among the physician, the patient, and the hospital organization during the patient's stay. This Patient's Bill of Rights could be included in the patient information booklet.

The admitting department also plays a major role in sustaining positive relations with the medical staff and hospital personnel. Indeed, all who come in contact with the department will form a reaction about the hospital based on their experience with the admitting staff. Many hospitals have initiated patient representative programs. Much of the work of the patient representatives encompasses the admitting department's functions. For example, patient representatives get involved in preadmission processing, credit arrangements, and patient discharge matters.

TYPES OF ADMISSIONS

In hospitals with a shortage of beds and a long waiting list, the categories or classifications of patients to be admitted are very important to the efficient functioning of the hospital. It has been common practice in hospitals to classify admissions based on the patient's medical needs. Of course, when there is a waiting list, the patient with the greatest medical need is generally admitted first.

Emergency admissions are patients who have to be immediately admitted to the hospital for the sake of their life or well-being. When there is not a vacant inpatient bed, emergency admissions could be housed in the hospital's emergency department's holding area. If absolutely necessary, the patient could also be housed in the nursing unit solarium or even in the patient unit corridor. The next category of admission is *urgent*. These patients must be admitted within 48 hours because their life or well-being could be threatened. The least critical category for admissions is *elective*. These patients' lives are not endangered if their admission is delayed. Under crowded conditions, elective patients generally go on a waiting list. It is common for the hospital's medical staff to be asked to review or to modify these admission definitions. Also the hospital's medical staff has an obligation to review the categories of admission and define them based on local community conditions, for example, by considering the age of the population and the services available in the hospital.

UTILIZATION REVIEW

With the passage of Public Law 92-603, which created the Professional Standards Review Organization (PSRO), the functions of the admissions office have been made more complex. The PSRO legislation provides for the monitoring of the quality and the appropriateness of hospital care rendered to Medicare and Medicaid patients. The government's intent is to reimburse hospitals only for hospital stays that are appropriate and required. This is a sensible objective. However, in practice it requires a great deal of clerical investigation by the hospital to determine whether the admission is clinically appropriate. Admitting physicians have to justify each patient's admission by providing a principal and secondary admission diagnosis. Based on this information, clinical criteria and a patient's probable length of stay can be reviewed. The admitting department's staff must understand its role in complying with the PSRO legislation. It has become mandatory for the staff to familiarize itself with the local PSRO admitting criteria and standards.

PREADMISSION

Admission of a patient can be facilitated if certain tasks are handled prior to the patient being admitted to the hospital. The preadmission process involves the admission's officer receiving pertinent patient data with the patient's hospital reservation. These data can be obtained days in advance of the patient's actual admission. The objective of gathering preadmission data is to expedite the processing of the patients into the hospital, thereby reducing waiting time in the admissions office or the lobby.

Preadmitting also allows for more efficient scheduling of patients into the inpatient area. To accomplish this objective, the admissions office generally sends the patient certain forms in advance to be completed and to be returned to the hospital prior to admission. The forms request the patient's name, address, certain statistical information, and details on the patient's financial insurance coverage. They also often ask if the patient has special requests, for example, a specific room accommodation or any special needs during the hospitalization.

Prior to the patient's admission, certain clinical preadmission testing is conducted on many elective patients. Third party payers concerned with the high cost of medical care encourage this preadmission testing process. The process of preadmission clinical testing involves the patient coming to the hospital for ancillary studies, including laboratory tests, x-ray examinations, or electrocardiograms. Testing generally is done on an outpatient basis prior to the day of admission. The majority of these tests turn out to be normal, or at least what the ordering physician expected. However, if an abnormality is discovered, the test results might delay a patient's surgery or at least his course of treatment. Under these circumstances, the patient might have to remain in the hospital longer than necessary. The patient may remain an outpatient until the particular problem is handled and can then enter the hospital for surgery.

Preadmission testing has four recognized benefits for the patient, the physician, and the hospital:

1. It frequently reduces the need to postpone or cancel surgery by discovering unusual test results prior to admission.
2. It allows the hospital's busy ancillary areas (x-ray and laboratory) to distribute the workload more evenly.
3. It provides information to the physician prior to the admission and makes the physician's preoperative patient workup much easier.
4. Since the testing is done on an outpatient basis, it frequently shortens the length of the patient's hospital stay; it thereby reduces the cost to the patient and to the insurance company and also frees beds for other patients.

Preadmission testing does have some drawbacks. Sometimes the patient is too ill to go to the hospital for diagnostic studies. Obviously, preadmission will not work on emergency admissions. Some patients are unwilling or unable to leave work or to go to the hospital a day or two prior to admission. Some patients find it inconvenient to travel long distances to the hospital. The Blue Cross insurance plans of this country have been the national leaders in preadmission testing.

On the other hand, the Blue Cross plans and Medicare are looking very critically at unnecessary diagnostic admission procedures. It has been common for hospitals to give patients a battery of tests—such as chest x-ray, electrocardiogram, and selected chemistry studies—prior to the patient's admission. Medicare's position on routine admission studies is that

> . . . "chest" x-rays, and other diagnostic procedures performed as part of the admitting procedure to a hospital should be specifically ordered by a physician and they should be found medically necessary for the diagnosis or treatment of the illness that the patient admitted to the hospital in order to be covered. Coverage of tests routinely performed [upon a doctor's standing orders] on admission could not, therefore, generally be considered reasonable and necessary. In addition, coverage of an admission test ordered by a physician should be questioned if it is known that the same test has been performed as part of an outpatient diagnostic workup prior to admission or in connection with a recent prior admission.[1]

One benefit of the preadmission testing program is the easing of the scheduling problems in the surgical suite. Operating room time must be scheduled in advance for patients who are admitted for elective surgery. With preadmission tests already accomplished before the patient is admitted, the operating room staff can better schedule its workload. The admitting department must work very closely with the operating room scheduler to coordinate the admission and the operating room time. Some hospitals allow the admitting department to schedule surgical time in the operating room, but this is not a common practice.

CONSENT FORMS

Frequently, the admitting department is responsible for obtaining a patient's signature on certain consent forms upon admission. Consent forms generally fall into two categories: (1) consent forms for general procedures and general treatment, and (2) special consent forms for any surgical or medical procedure. Usually the admitting officer is responsible for the general consent forms, while the physicians and other clinical members of the medical team may be involved in obtaining signatures on the special consent forms, since they require informed consent. General consent forms often cover routine procedures such as laboratory work, x-rays, or simple medical treatment. Special consent forms are involved in major or minor surgery, anesthesia, cobalt or certain x-ray treatments, and experimental procedures.

BED ASSIGNMENTS

The matter of assigning patients to beds is usually a problem only when a hospital has high occupancies or a waiting list. When the hospital has empty beds, the assignments are generally on a "first come-first served" basis. When a hospital has high occupancies or waiting lists, frustration levels among patients, physicians, and the admitting office staff run high. Therefore, it is necessary for the hospital to have an admission's policy and a scheduling procedure.

Establishment of the specific policies and procedures is up to the individual hospital in concert with its medical staff. However, some criteria that are used include: (1) maximizing occupancy; (2) clinical segregation of patients (more often done in teaching or university hospitals), which allows the medical department, the surgical department, and other specialty areas to receive a reasonable balance of patients in the hospital; (3) minimizing the bad debts or maximizing revenue or income; and (4) allotting certain hospital beds for teaching cases (frequently seen in medical teaching centers where it is used to maximize the teaching cases for residents and medical students).

If the hospital fails to utilize its beds properly and to employ a reasonable policy and procedure for allocation, it will only serve to drive up the cost per patient day, since empty beds add to the cost and force a hospital to operate at less than maximum efficiency. This is the principal reason that management should be concerned with a bed allocation policy.

NOTE

1. Medicare Bulletin, 79-34, November 2, 1979, AETNA Life Insurance Company, Medicare Administration. Hospital Admission and Diagnostic Procedures which are defined as "reasonable and necessary" and therefore covered under Medicare relate to Section 1862(a)(1) of the act and Section 405-310(k) of the Medicare regulations.

Part IV

The Medical Team

Chapter 9

The Medical Staff

Key Terms

Allied medical staff ⁓ National Internship Matching Plan ⁓ Approved residency program ⁓ Chief resident ⁓ Specialty boards ⁓ American Medical Association (AMA) ⁓ Association of American Medical Colleges (AAMC) ⁓ Council on Medical Education & Hospitals of the AMA ⁓ Appointment process ⁓ Credentials committee ⁓ Categories of membership ⁓ Departmental organization ⁓ Department chairman ⁓ Executive committee ⁓ Clinical privileges ⁓ Joint Conference Committee (JCC)

INTRODUCTION

The medical staff has the greatest impact on the quality and quantity of care given in the hospital. The medical staff is the heart of the hospital. The members of the staff render the medical care to the patients. Though the governing body has the ultimate legal and moral responsibility for the hospital, including the quality of medical care, the board of trustees cannot practice medicine and is dependent upon the members of the medical staff to admit patients and to provide quality patient care.

The medical staff is appointed by the board of trustees. The staff is then expected to formulate its own medical policies, rules, and regulations and to be responsible to the board for the quality of patient care. Though the medical profession is a highly disciplined, professional group, it is made up of highly individualistic members who have their own unique approaches to medicine and organizational relationships. Therefore, the task of coordinating the efforts of the medical staff with the board of trustees, the administrator, and the rest of the hospital can be a challenging one.

WHAT IS THE MEDICAL STAFF?

The hospital medical staff is an organized body of physicians, dentists, perhaps podiatrists, and in some instances an allied medical staff professional who attends patients and participates in related duties with patient care. Members of the medical staff have been authorized by the board of trustees to attend patients in the hospital and are accountable to the governing authority. They are accountable to the hospital for high-quality patient care through the application of ethical, clinical, and scientific procedures and practices. The majority of the members of the medical staff are physicians; this is a JCAH requirement. There are an estimated 380,000 physicians in this country, many of whom practice on hospital staffs.

BECOMING A PHYSICIAN

The training period to become a doctor is a long and arduous one. In the 1950s and 1960s, it included at least four years of undergraduate school to earn a bachelor's degree, four years of medical school, and another six to eight years of internship and residency. Often military service had to be served. Then the physician had to spend some period of time in the practice of medicine before becoming certified in a specialty.

Despite the recent efforts of a few medical schools to shorten the required 4-year curriculum, it is still virtually impossible for a physician to start practice before 9 to 11 years of education beyond high school. The residency requirements for specialty training continue to lengthen. For the most part, physicians will be approximately 30 years old before they are out on their own practicing medicine. After graduating from medical school, most graduates look to passing a state licensing examination. Records show that most graduates of medical schools in the United States pass state licensing examinations on their first try.[1] The vast majority of graduates also go on to postgraduate or residency training. Entering medical school is a highly competitive business. There are 126 medical schools in the United States. There are approximately 350,000 applications made for only 14,800 actual positions.[2]

RESIDENCIES

After graduating from medical school, it is mandatory that a newly graduated physician seek a residency or postgraduate specialty training program in a hospital. This he does by applying for the National Internship Matching Plan; this is a scheme developed in July 1951 by representatives from the American Association of Medical Colleges, the AMA, and different hospital associations. This group acts as a national clearinghouse for matching the preferences of the individual graduating medical students and the hospitals offering residencies.

The clearinghouse function gives a greater degree of freedom of choice for both the hospital and the student. Before the matching plan, graduating students from medical schools had to negotiate their own internship or residency with individual hospitals. Since the students were notified by a specific date, it was often too late in the year to seek alternate internships if they were turned down. The matching plan allows for more students to be placed in approved residency programs (approved by the Council of Education). Before the Millis Report, internships were predominantly the first year's postgraduate training for physicians. However, the internship category has now been eliminated, and the first year is called the first year of residency. The matching plan has shown that an average of approximately 96 percent of the students are matched each year.[3]

A hospital that has an approved residency program is more complex, and perhaps more interesting, than a hospital that does not offer programs for educating physicians. There are some 1,267 hospitals in the country that have American Medical Association (AMA) or American Osteopathic Association (AOA) approved residencies with 31,502 residents in training.

Currently, there are 22 different specialty residency programs available. The teaching hospital is essentially a living classroom. In these hospitals, the residents are considered vital members of the house staff. The students' excitement for fresh ideas in medicine and their zest for knowledge enliven the entire atmosphere of the hospital. Generally, these first-year residents are not licensed physicians, though in many states special temporary licenses are granted to practice within the institution that has the approved residency program. These residents are not independent contractors but are considered hospital employees. There was a time when the residents worked for a meager stipend. Now the residents receive respectable salaries for their efforts. The residents gain much from the hospital but also give the hospital a great deal in patient service, though their service role may at times conflict with their goals as students and learners.

Residents in a hospital pose a complicated organizational problem. They are essentially employees of the hospital, but they are doing medical staff work. The residency program is a hierarchical organization, just like many other departments within the hospital. First-year residents are the low persons on the totem pole; they are under the guidance of a senior resident who in turn is under the guidance of the head or chief resident of a given specialty. The chief residents in each specialty have the supervisory, managerial, and teaching responsibilities in the program. Generally, the nursing department and the residents get along well together, working as partners for the most part.

After physicians complete their hospital residency programs, they seek to become certified in their specialties. Certification is under the jurisdiction of specialty boards, such as the American Board of Surgery. Specialty associations,

such as The American College of Surgeons, also have considerable influence on
the newly graduated specialists.

The objective of specialty boards and associations is to upgrade the qualifications of specialists. These boards and associations have increased the length of
time needed for training, developed subspecialties, and sponsored numerous
continuing education programs and professional journals. After rigorous examinations and proven abilities and practice, certification by a specialty board is indeed a
recognition of professional competency. Fellowship in a specialty college is also a
meaningful peer recognition of competence.

Specialty groups have come under criticism for their inattention to national
manpower requirements.[4] Nonetheless, because of the efforts of these specialty
boards, today's graduates from American medical schools with board training and
board certification are better trained physicians.

ORGANIZED MEDICINE

In 1847, some 250 physicians, representing more than 40 medical societies and
28 colleges from 22 states, came together and founded the American Medical
Association (AMA).[5] Pressure to begin the AMA stemmed from the poor quality
of medical education in the United States at that time, the very brisk traffic in
patent medicines and secret remedies, and the questionable ethics of many physicians of the time. The men who founded the AMA believed that a national
association of physicians was needed to lead the crusade for improved medical
education and patient care. The founding objectives of the AMA are two-fold:
(1) to "promote the science and art of medicine and the betterment of public
health," and (2) to promote "better health for all people and service to the
professional needs of its membership."[6]

Membership in the AMA is open to any physician who has good standing in the
local medical society. The AMA is a federation of some 54 constituent medical
associations. These associations are in turn composed of more than 1,900 medical
societies. Perhaps one of the AMA's greatest contributions to medicine is its
"systematic and continuing gathering of data on new products, new findings, and
new methods. This information is correlated, evaluated, summarized and chan-
neled to the AMA members."[7]

More recently, the AMA has become more and more involved in the legislative
process and has become a part of a strong hospital and medical lobby. One of the
long-standing criticisms of the AMA is that it has exerted too much influence over
the accreditation of medical schools. Accreditation is actually done through the
AMA's Association of American Medical Colleges (AAMC).

On December 11, 1978, the Federal Trade Commission (FTC) accused the AMA
of exerting too much influence over medical schools. The FTC has contended

that the "AMA and AAMC" are not autonomous in accordance with governmental regulations."[8] Not surprisingly, the AMA responded by indicating that this was simply "another case of government intervention into professional affairs."[9] A man outside the medical area who would agree with the Federal Trade Commission is the outstanding economist, Milton Friedman. In his classic text, *Capitalism and Freedom,* he wrote a provocative discourse on medical licensure. Friedman holds the position that the AMA, as a trade union, has limited the number of people who can enter the union or the medical profession. He points out that the Council on Medical Education and Hospitals of the AMA is the body that approves medical schools and that this council is controlled in part by the AMA. He indicates that control over admission to medical schools and later licensure has enabled the AMA to limit entry into its profession in two ways: (1) by simply turning down many applicants to medical school, and (2) by establishing standards for admissions and licensure that make entry so difficult as to discourage young people from ever getting admitted to the schools.[10]

MEDICAL STAFF ORGANIZATION

The internal organization of the medical staff will vary from hospital to hospital. The more complex, university teaching hospitals will differ from the smaller community hospitals. The differences are less today because of the efforts of the JCAH and its accreditation standards. These standards stipulate that "there shall be a single organized medical staff that has the overall responsibility for the quality of all medical care provided to patients, and for the ethical conduct in professional practices of its members, as well as for accounting therefore to the governing body."[11]

Appointment to the medical staff is a formal process that is outlined in each medical staff's bylaws, again with encouragement for standardization from the JCAH. A brief outline of the appointment process that a doctor must go through is as follows:

- The applying physician completes a written application and forwards it to the governing body, usually through the hospital CEO.

- The application is reviewed for completeness and verification and then sent to the head of the department to which the applicant is applying for initial quality screening.

- The application is then forwarded to the medical staff's credentials committee, which reviews the qualifications and past professional performance of the physician. It is at this point that the physician generally makes a personal appearance before the doctors on the credentials committee.

- The executive committee of the medical staff reviews the application and gives its concurrence.

- The medical staff gives its written recommendation to the hospital governing body.

- The board of trustees either accepts, rejects, or defers the application. If the application is questionable and needs discussion, it may be referred to the joint conference committee.

- The physician is notified by the CEO or the secretary of the governing body that the appointment has been approved or disapproved and with what limitations on privileges.

The physician who has applied and has been admitted to the staff is appointed in two separate categories of membership: (1) to a special clinical area of a department, and (2) with a status based on the extent of the physician's participation and privileges. The status that the physician is assigned could be one of "active" medical staff, "courtesy" medical staff, or "consulting" medical staff. The differences between these categories usually revolve around the extent to which the physician wants to be active in a given hospital. Active status includes full rights and privileges, voting prerogatives, and obligations to attend meetings, serve on committees, and handle emergency service responsibilities. Courtesy and consulting physicians have fewer privileges and responsibilities.

The organization of the hospital staff is divided into medical specialty departments. For example, there are departments of medicine, surgery, obstetrics and gynecology, and pediatrics. In larger hospitals, these departments may be further subdivided. Each clinical department has a chief or chairperson who is the medical administrative head. This person is generally selected through a process outlined in the medical staff bylaws. Usually this is done either through election by departmental members or by appointment by the hospital.

In applying for membership, a physician is granted certain clinical privileges (procedures the physician is permitted to perform within the hospital). This process is referred to as privilege delineation. The privilege delineation process is based on verifiable information made available to the credentials committee. Privileges should be based on a physician's demonstrated current competence in a discipline. The privileges are listed on a delineation-of-privileges form and kept on file in key places within the hospital—for example, within the operating room and the administrator's office.

CLOSED AND OPEN MEDICAL STAFFS

Historically, individual hospitals have controlled their own admissions to medical staff. However, in recent years hospitals' autonomy has eroded in this area. A closed medical staff is one that closely monitors and restricts any new applicants to the staff or to a department of the staff. This is generally done with the concurrence of the hospital board of trustees. When a hospital does permit a closed medical staff, it is usually based upon considerations related to the quality of patient care. There may also be closed medical staffs within selected departments in the hospital—the two most notable examples are the radiology department and the pathology department. In these departments the hospital signs an agreement with one physician or one professional group to provide exclusive services in the department. The courts have generally found this to be a legal arrangement if such agreements are based upon significant medical and administrative considerations. Closed medical staff issues are constantly being addressed in the courts under the Federal Anti-Trust Laws. Additionally, since the Federal Trade Commission (FTC) has the power to promulgate rules and regulations defining unfair practices in this area, it is reasonable to assume that it will be a predominant enforcement agency relative to medical staff admission in years to come.

THE MEDICAL DIRECTOR

For several years there has been a trend for boards and administrators to employ full-time medical directors. Management apparently feels this is the best way to fulfill its responsibility for quality care. Not surprisingly, medical staffs often see this trend as a threat to their self-governance. The medical director is a member of hospital management and, even though he or she may be a member of the medical staff, answers to the administrator. The medical director's role is primarily to evaluate clinical performance and to enforce hospital policy related to quality care.

MEDICAL STAFF BYLAWS, RULES, AND REGULATIONS

JCAH standards dictate that "the medical staff shall develop and adopt bylaws, rules, and regulations to establish a framework of self-government and a means for accountability to the governing body."[12] The bylaws outline the form of self-government of the medical staff. The medical staff conducts its business through committees. The committee chairpersons are either selected by members of the staff or appointed by the president of the staff.

One of the most important committees is the medical staff executive committee. It continues the medical staff business in the interim between general staff meetings. This committee is usually composed of the officers of the staff and a number of elected members from the staff. Typically, the medical executive committee meets once a month to keep abreast of the business of the medical staff and to relate to the management of the hospital. Generally, the medical executive committee coordinates the policies of the various clinical department staffs.

Other crucial committees of the medical staff include the credentials committee, the medical records committee, the tissue committee, and the medical audit committee.

The credentials committee is charged with the responsibility to review the qualifications of physicians applying to the medical staff. It also reviews the credentials of the medical staff members who must be reappointed once or twice every two years. Occasionally, the credentials committee might be asked to investigate breaches of ethics or misconduct among the members of the medical staff. This committee reports directly to the executive committee.

Since medical records have now become the instrument for review of quality assurance programs and medical audits, the medical records committee has taken on a more important function in recent years. Initially, it was responsible for reviewing the forms that could be used in the medical records. It now also reviews the quantity and quality of the patient records as written by the physicians and other associated health professionals in the hospital. It also serves as a monitor on the physicians who may have delinquent medical records. This committee has the closest working relationship with the hospital's medical records administrator.

One of the traditional methods of conducting a hospital and medical audit has been a well-functioning tissue committee. This committee provides a medium to confirm the diagnosis for surgical cases and acts as the monitor on unnecessary surgery. The tissue committee usually consists of practicing surgeons plus a member of the hospital pathology department. The tissue committee reviews all surgical cases to determine, based on the review of tissue taken from the patient, whether the operation was in fact necessary. It is the custom for each surgeon who removes tissue from an operation to forward this to the pathology laboratory for postoperative diagnosis.

The medical audit committee also guards quality assurance in the hospital. This committee is a group of physicians who review the practice of medicine in all disciplines—medical, surgical, obstetrics, gynecology, and pediatrics. Attention is given to the progress notes, the clinical course of the patient, the kinds of treatment rendered patients, and the outcome of the treatment. Since the inception of Medicare in 1966, the medical audit committee has been joined by the utilization review committee; together they form the quality assurance committee in most hospitals.

The Joint Conference Committee (JCC) consists of members of the medical staff, frequently representatives from the executive committee, who meet with representatives from the administration and the board of trustees. The JCC is the forum for the three major power groups to discuss medical staff problems and issues. It is not, however, generally a decision-making body but usually refers its recommendations and deliberations to the board of trustees.

CONTINUING MEDICAL EDUCATION

Following appointment to the medical staff of the hospital, the physician is obligated to provide proof of participation in a program of continuing medical education (CME). In fact, JCAH standards stipulate that "the medical staff shall participate in a program of continuing education."[13] The scope and complexity of a physician's individual continuing education program or the hospital's program are left to each institution. It will vary depending on the resources at hand and the needs of the hospital. However, a hospital program must be relevant to the type of patient care delivered at the hospital. When a hospital does participate in a program, each staff member's participation should be documented and placed in that member's medical staff file.

The courts have determined that the governing body has the ultimate legal responsibility for the quality of medical care practiced in a hospital; but it rests with the medical staff (who are appointed by the board of trustees) to formulate the proper medical policies, to have them approved by the board of trustees, and to carry out the quality of patient care according to the highest possible professional standards. The medical staff organization is unique within the hospital since it is allowed to discipline itself. Medical staffs operate best when they are thoroughly organized and relate in a positive way both with the administration and the governing body of the hospital.

ALLIED HEALTH PERSONNEL

Over the last ten years there have been an increasing number of nonphysicians and nondentists applying for clinical privileges within the hospital, including but not limited to podiatrists, chiropractors, physician assistants, nurse practitioners, and nurse midwives. By applying for medical staff privileges, some of these groups have raised the question of how they fit into the hospital medical staff.

Historically, with the backing of laws and regulations, hospitals have excluded these groups from practicing within the hospital. Generally, state regulations regarding nurse practitioners and physician assistants indicate that a physician must supervise their work. The American Medical Association basically agrees with the American Hospital Association on this issue and feels that full medical staff privileges should be restricted to physicians and dentists. The Joint Commission on Accreditation of Hospitals has been somewhat more liberal with regard to podiatrists and has delineated what it believes a podiatrist can do within a hospital. The JCAH permits other duly licensed health care professionals to practice in hospitals under the supervision of a practitioner who has clinical privileges. The case law on the privilege question is not absolutely clear, and it is reasonable to assume that each individual issue may be decided based upon state statutes and license practice laws within that state.

NOTES

1. Rockwell Schulz and Alton C. Johnson, *Management of Hospitals* (New York, N.Y.: McGraw-Hill Book Co., 1976), p. 71.

2. Ibid., p. 69.

3. Robert M. Farrier, "National Intern Resident Matching Program," *Hospital Progress,* November 1973, p. 12.

4. Schulz and Johnson, *Management of Hospitals,* p. 74.

5. Leslie J. DeGroot, *Medical Care: Social and Organizationing Aspects* (Springfield, Ill.: Charles C. Thomas, 1966), p. 438.

6. Ibid.

7. Ibid., p. 442.

8. American Hospital Association, *Hospital Week* (Chicago, December 1978), Vol. 14, No. 49.

9. Ibid.

10. Milton Friedman, *Capitalism and Freedom* (Chicago, Ill.: University of Chicago Press, 1972), p. 151.

11. Joint Commission on Accreditation of Hospitals, *Accreditation Manual for Hospitals-1980 Edition* (Chicago, Ill., 1979), p. 93.

12. Ibid., p. 103.

13. Ibid., p. 108.

Nursing Services

Key Terms

Mother of modern nursing ⌁ Nursing service director ⌁ Nursing supervisor ⌁ Nursing school ⌁ Head nurse ⌁ Staff nurse ⌁ State nursing board ⌁ Auxiliary nursing personnel ⌁ Nursing unit ⌁ Nurses' station ⌁ American Nurses Associa-. tion (ANA) ⌁ National League for Nursing (NLN) ⌁ Nursing standard ⌁ Master plan ⌁ Case nursing ⌁ Functional nursing ⌁ Team nursing ⌁ Primary care nursing ⌁ Cyclical scheduling ⌁ Clinical nurse specialist ⌁ Nurse clinician ⌁ Nurse practitioners ⌁ Nurse midwife ⌁ Intensive care unit (ICU) ⌁ Coronary care unit (CCU) ⌁ Patient monitoring

INTRODUCTION

Hospitalized patients should receive gentle, courteous, and considerate care given by skillful, understanding personnel. The primary department to meet this goal is the nursing service department. Nurses account for the single largest health professional group in the country. In 1977, there were 1,409,434 professional nurses of whom 988,050 were employed in nursing. Of this large number, approximately 63 percent were employed in hospitals. At the same time, there were approximately 360,000 medical doctors. Since the nursing service department accounts for 25 percent of all hospital operating expenses and represents 36 to 37 percent of total hospital salary expenses and employees, it is a major factor in the hospital.[1a and b]

EARLY TRADITIONS

Early organized nursing services began under the auspices of Roman Catholic sisters who dedicated their lives to nursing. There were also notable individuals who contributed to the early traditions of nursing. The religious influence, the authoritative influence of individuals, and the nursing traditions established by the military were the three major influences that impacted the early history of nursing.

Perhaps the best known person associated with the history of nursing is Florence Nightingale, whose work in the Crimea with the British soldiers brought her public recognition. She became known as the "mother of modern nursing." Florence Nightingale established and founded the Florence Nightingale Nursing School in connection with St. Thomas Hospital in London in 1859.[2]

Schools for training nurses in America can be found as far back as 1798. However, schools that really embodied the principles of Florence Nightingale's school in London were established in the United States much later. The first such school was the New England Hospital for Women and Children founded in Boston in 1872. This was followed in 1873 by the Bellevue Hospital School of Nursing in New York City. The Massachusetts General Hospital in Boston opened its school of nursing in 1873 also. Over the next 50 years, there were some 2,000 nursing schools established in the United States.[3] Today, there are 1,765 nursing schools in the United States. These schools' programs include practical nursing school programs, diploma programs based in hospitals, two-year associate degree programs in junior colleges and colleges, and four-year baccalaureate programs in colleges and universities. Table 10-1 outlines the educational requirements for nurses.

DEPARTMENT ORGANIZATION

Approximately 50 percent of all employees in a hospital work in the nursing service department. Each of the many varied positions in the department has a job description. In each hospital, the department must have specific job descriptions and procedure manuals.

The nursing service department is organized in a pyramid fashion very much like the hospital as a whole. The primary responsibility rests with the director of the nursing service department, referred to as the director of nurses (DON). These directors are usually selected because of their management abilities; they are often registered nurses with advanced degrees (sometimes in the specific discipline of nursing service administration). Often, the director has one or two assistant directors to aid in the management of the department. The title of supervisor is frequently given to the position held by a registered nurse who supervises or directs the activities of two or more nursing units. The supervisor may manage and direct the many nursing service activities during the evenings, nights, or weekends; thus, the titles of night supervisor, weekend supervisor, or day supervisor are often applied. If a hospital has a nursing school, the director of nursing is often responsible for both the nursing service and the nursing school. Or the nursing school may have its own director who reports to the director of nurses. If there is no

Table 10-1 Educational Requirements for Nurses

Educational Level	Training Required beyond High School	Curriculum	Training Site
Registered nurse— Ph.D. and D.N.S. (Doctor of Nursing Science)	3 to 5 years post-baccalaureate	Academic program integrated with practical work throughout the years	University
Registered nurse— master's degree	5 to 6 academic years	1 to 2 year academic program integrated with practical work	University, hospital and community health agencies
Registered nurse— baccalaureate degree	4 years and summer sessions	4-year academic program integrated with practical experience	University, hospital and community health agencies
Registered nurse— diploma	27-36 months	1 year academic work, 2 years of practical experience with clinical courses	Hospital
Registered nurse— associate degree	2 years	2-year academic program integrated with practical experience	Junior college
Licensed practical nurse (LPN)	1 year	1-year academic program integrated with practical experience	Vocational technical school and hospital

school of nursing, the training function of the nursing department is usually assigned to an assistant director who is responsible for the education, orientation, and continuing inservice education of all employees in the department of nursing.

The nursing service department is also organized along geographical lines. Each of the nursing service responsibilities for patient care is decentralized to a specific location in the hospital called a nursing unit or patient care unit. Certain responsibilities and functions to operate a nursing unit are assigned to a head nurse. A head nurse supervises the personnel in a patient care unit. This person is accountable for the quality of the nursing care on the unit, controls the supplies, and schedules the staff. Usually the head nurse has a series of staff nurses. In some cases, the porters and maids report to the head nurse, although this is not common. The majority of nurses who work under a head nurse are called staff nurses or general duty nurses. The staff nurses are assigned specific responsibilities for the nursing care of patients on the nursing unit.

There have been an increasing number of practical nurses (PN) or licensed graduate practical nurses (LGPN) entering the nursing scene over the last several years. Practical nurses are trained in a formal LGPN program in a hospital or vocational school. Generally, the program covers a formal one-year training period. After the formal education, the practical nurse takes a state nursing board examination to be licensed.

A large number of employees in the nursing service are grouped under the title of auxiliary nursing personnel; these include nurse aides, attendants, nursing technicians, and orderlies. Auxiliary nursing personnel generally go through a hospital orientation training program before assuming their nursing duties with patients. They do not need to be graduates of a formal educational program, nor are they licensed or certified. These personnel generally are assigned duties by the graduate nurse, staff nurse, or head nurse.

Many of the individual nursing units have a host of clerical functions to be performed. The clerks assigned to nursing service handle the huge quantity of paperwork, answer telephones, direct visitors, help with hospital requisitions for patients and supplies, and perform other similar duties. These clerks usually work directly under the supervision of a head nurse.

THE NURSING UNIT

As noted earlier, the nursing care of the hospital is organized in a decentralized fashion into patient care units or nursing units. The size of nursing units varies. They can be very small, with 8- to 10-bed units for specialized care, or they can be large, with 60- to 70-bed units. Perhaps the most common size is between 20 and 40 beds per unit.[4] Nursing units operate on three shifts to cover the 24-hour period. They generally operate as a day shift between 7:00 A.M. and 3:00 P.M. The evening shift, called the evening tour, runs from 3:00 P.M. to 11:00 P.M., and the night shift from 11:00 P.M. to 7:00 A.M.

There are disagreements over the most effective way to organize the distribution of patient rooms on a nursing unit. Most rooms are semiprivate or multibed accommodations, with two, three, four, or even up to six beds in one room. More recently, there has been a trend toward the private or single-bed accommodation. Studies on efficiency and effectiveness, comparing the private room to the multi-patient accommodation, are still being evaluated.

The size of the nursing unit and the distribution of single and multibed rooms are considered before a unit is built. Consideration is given to the cost of construction of the unit, the duplication of equipment, and how much nursing service time will be required to staff the unit. If the unit is spacious and rooms are distributed a distance from the central nursing point, the staff must continually travel to reach a patient and supplies. Although the unit may look pleasing, it may not be efficient to work in. There are a variety of designs and configurations for nursing units. Some of the more common nursing unit layouts are shown in Exhibit 10-1.

PATIENT ROOMS

Whether the patient rooms are private or multi-accommodations, they will vary in size. It has been suggested that the minimum size for a private room should be not less than 125 square feet with a minimum width of at least 12 feet, 6 inches.[5] As to the two-bed accommodation, a minimum of 160 square feet is usually provided with the beds separated by cubicle curtains. For a four-bed room, the minimum is generally considered to be 320 square feet. The hospital bed is generally 86 inches long, 36 inches wide, about 27 inches from the floor, and can be varied electrically or mechanically into different positions.

OTHER COMPONENTS OF THE NURSING UNIT

Among the elements found on nursing units is the nurses' station, which tends to be the focal point of administrative activity. The nurses' station is generally where the nurses keep their records and is centrally located to all the activities of the entire nursing unit. On a nursing unit there is also a medicine preparation room area. Every nursing unit has a utility room. This is a work space where clean supplies, instruments, and equipment and "used" or "dirty" equipment that has been used by the patients are stored. Usually there is also a small pantry, or sometimes even a large kitchen, on the nursing unit, depending on the method used by the hospital to deliver its dietary services. If the food is prepackaged or preplated before coming to the nursing unit, a smaller pantry will suffice. If the

Exhibit 10-1 Various Shapes of Floor Plans with Alternative Designs

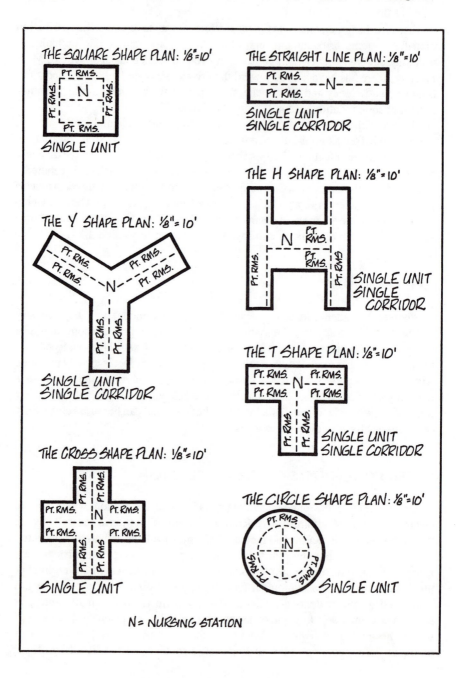

food is delivered to the nursing unit in bulk fashion and distributed, there may be a need for a larger kitchen.

Other rooms that might be found on nursing units are a common toilet/bath area (if they are not available individually in the patient rooms), a consultation room where physicians and the families of the patients may meet, and treatment rooms. Some units may also have a pleasant place for visitors to sit down with the patients outside of their rooms.

NURSING EDUCATION

Profound changes in the well-established Florence Nightingale nursing education model emerged following World War II. With the acute shortages of registered professional nurses during the war, the licensed practical nurse (LPN) came more into vogue. The number of nurse aides continued to expand rapidly up until the mid-1970s. Meanwhile, the registered nurse educational programs had begun to change, especially in the 1960s. During this time, the three-year, hospital-diploma, nursing education programs began to be phased out because of the high cost of nursing education and pressures from the American Nurses Association for a baccalaureate or associate degree education.[6]

Registered nurses can earn a Ph.D., which usually takes more than seven years of academic work. A nurse with a master's degree will have spent five to six years in college, while a baccalaureate registered nurse will have studied for four years. Usually, the diploma registered nurse goes to school from 27 to 36 months in a hospital, while the two-year associate degree registered nurse is a graduate from a junior college (see Table 10-1).

There are two large and influential professional nursing association groups. The American Nurses Association (ANA) is a federation of 54 constituent associations, including those in the 50 states, the District of Columbia, and Puerto Rico. As a group they promote legislation and speak out for nurses on legislative action programs. The other influential nursing association is the National League for Nursing (NLN). This is a community-centered group that brings together people in the health and welfare fields with the lay community to work primarily for the improvement of nursing service and nursing education. The NLN's membership is composed of registered nurses, practical nurses, nurse aides, doctors, and hospital administrators—all with a professional interest in nursing. The NLN began in 1952 with the merger of seven national nursing organizations and national committees. The League's structure indicates its major program interests. Some of these are hospital nursing, public health nursing, public service departments, and better baccalaureate and higher degree programs, as well as diploma and associate degree programs, of education. Perhaps the diversity of the NLN membership is one of the main differences between the ANA and NLN

TERMS AND STANDARDS

An understanding of precisely which nursing standard was used when the nursing department's budget and staffing schedule were established is an important element in nursing service. A nursing standard or nursing norm is defined as the amount of time and resources needed or considered desirable for each patient in a 24-hour period in order to give the type of care judged appropriate. (The American Hospital Association and the National League for Nursing identified various nursing standards in 1950.) Nursing managers should be able to ask such questions as: Is the ratio of registered nurses to other personnel in the department too high? Are there too many or too few licensed practical nurses for the situation? Is there another way to assign duties in order to improve budgetary performance?

Financial managers should know that when nursing service expenses are low or below budget, a detailed look at the nursing staff patterns may be required. Perhaps student nurses have been utilized in place of staff nurses. Perhaps private duty nurses were attached to some other cost center and were used in place of regular staff nurses. Perhaps inadequate information was available at the time the budget was established. Perhaps the department was unable to fill all budgeted positions. Perhaps the onduty nursing staff is carrying an unfair load. To analyze all these specific circumstances, a financial manager must have an understanding of certain nursing definitions and terms that are widely accepted in the nursing service area.

The patient, upon entering the hospital, in effect agrees to an unwritten contract that the care the hospital renders will be adequate. The questions are: What is adequate care? How many registered nurses and ancillary nursing staff are required to provide adequate care? These are important questions that are central to the nursing department's mission. They should be answered and evaluated only in the light of a nursing standard.[7]

STAFFING

Nurse staffing is the result of determining the appropriate number of full-time equivalent nursing personnel (FTEs) by each nursing skill class (RNs, LPNs, nurse aides) to properly operate each nursing unit. This should be done prior to budget preparation. Daily, weekly, and seasonal variations must be considered. Through the consideration of these variations, it is appropriate to identify the number of "float" nurses and part-time nursing pool personnel who will be necessary to meet peak census periods on the nursing unit.

Historically, there have been many patterns used to staff nursing units.[8] Today there tend to be four commonly used modes: case method of nursing, functional nursing, team nursing, and primary care nursing.

Case Nursing

The case method of nursing is one of the earliest forms of nursing care. In this system, the nurse individually plans and administers the care of a patient. This is done on a one-to-one basis. The case method has persisted over the years in a couple of nursing areas. It is used today as the model of nursing in nursing schools because it allows nursing students to be taught the "idealized" patient care system. It is also used in acute care settings, such as intensive care, and may be used on the general nursing unit in private duty nursing situations.

Functional Nursing

Starting in the 1920s and continuing into the 1940s, nurses became aware of the studies and developments in the functional division of labor in industry, as seen in the assembly line approach to manufacturing used by Henry Ford and other industrialists. Nurses then applied these time and motion studies to their own discipline. Essentially, functional nursing uses a pyramid organization to look at the division of labor. Under such an arrangement, each of the members of the nursing staff on the unit has technical aspects of that member's job identified; with this knowledge, each unit member is given specific functions or tasks to perform on the unit. For example, one nurse might administer medications, another would give all the treatments, a third might take all the temperatures and blood pressures of patients, and a fourth might prepare those patients going to surgery or x-ray. All would give baths, make beds, and try to meet the patient's psychological and emotional needs. The simpler tasks would be given to the less trained nursing personnel; the more complex tasks, to the registered nurse. Functional nursing is often utilized on the evening and night shifts where the number of tasks has generally been reduced.

Team Nursing

Team nursing began around World War II when there was a shortage of registered nurses (RNs). In the absence of RNs, hospitals had to use technicians, vocational nurses, and nurse aides. Frequently, the less trained nursing personnel were put under the supervision of a more highly trained registered nurse, who was called the team leader. This team was asked to provide care to a group of patients on the nursing unit. Ideally, the team leader was the best prepared person and was expected to facilitate the team in formulating and carrying out the nursing care plans for every patient assigned to the team. Team nursing fits very well into the pyramid structure of the hospital organization.

Primary Care Nursing

Primary care nursing has some of the characteristics of the case method of nursing, in that one registered nurse is assigned to each patient. However, unlike the case method of nursing, the nurse assigned to the patient is not responsible only for one shift of work. The primary care nurse is responsible for the care of the patient for 24 hours a day, 7 days a week. It is the primary care nurse's responsibility to assess a patient's nursing needs. The primary care nurse collaborates with other health professionals, including the physician, and formulates a plan of nursing care for which the nurse becomes responsible and accountable. The primary care nurse may delegate certain responsibilities for executing that plan on the other shifts, but the delegation is accomplished by means of other nursing care plans, including written notes and recordings. Carrying out the plan is never done through a supervisory or third party; thus an important element of primary care nursing is the "triple A nurse." The triple A nurse is *a*utonomous, has the *a*uthority, and is held *a*ccountable for the nursing care of the patient.

One of the management tools used by nursing administration to assign personnel efficiently to a unit is the patient classification system. "In nursing, the term patient classification means the categorization of patients according to some assessment of their nursing care requirements over a specified period of time."[9] Some hospitals use direct care sampling forms in conjunction with the patient assessment system to provide a basis for forecasting workload.

SCHEDULING

Once the nursing department agrees to the standards to be used to staff the nursing unit and the nursing administration agrees on the type of nursing (nursing modalities) best suited for the hospital, the challenge to nursing then is to schedule nursing personnel so that the patients receive the care at the time they require it. Nurse scheduling is defined as determining when each member of the nursing staff will be on duty and on which shift each will work. Scheduling should take into account weekends, length of an individual's work stretches, and nursing requests for vacation and time off. Scheduling is typically done for a period of four or six weeks, and the scheduling is frequently tailored to each individual nursing unit. There are three commonly used approaches to nurse scheduling: the traditional, the cyclical, and computer-aided traditional approaches.[10]

Traditional Scheduling

In traditional scheduling, the nurse schedulers start from scratch each period (week, month). Generally, the head nurse makes the scheduling decisions by taking pencil and paper in hand and looking at the roster of personnel who are available to work on specified dates and for certain durations. This places in the head nurse's hands a great deal of responsibility for the quality and quantity of coverage on the nursing unit. The major advantage of this traditional approach is its flexibility. Since nurses begin essentially from scratch each period, they are able to adjust to changes of environment on the nursing unit quite quickly. Some of traditional scheduling's disadvantages include spottiness in coverage at times and uneven quality of coverage. Unless policies in the nursing administration leave some flexibility in the process, uneven staffing could also lead to higher personnel cost.

Cyclical Scheduling

Cyclical scheduling is a system that covers a certain period of time, perhaps one or three months. This block of time is the cycle or scheduling period. Once having agreed on a definite period, the scheduling in the cycle simply repeats itself period after period. The advantage of cyclical scheduling is that it provides even coverage with a higher quality of coverage determined for each nursing unit. Special requests would interfere with the coverage, which could impact the quality of staffing. The major disadvantage to cyclical scheduling is that it is inflexible compared to the traditional system and is not able to adjust rapidly to changes in the nursing unit environment. The ability to adjust is important, since change characterizes so many nursing units. The environment in which cyclical scheduling seems to work best is one in which the number of patients and their needs are fairly constant and the nurses are stable and do not rotate between shifts. New nurses can be hired into any open cyclical slot with very little difficulty.

Computer-Aided Traditional Scheduling

The third approach to scheduling uses the computer to help the traditional method of scheduling. This permits mathematical programming to be applied to traditional nurse scheduling. This system provides the traditional approach with more flexibility, and it also reduces the operating costs involved in calculating and in working with the schedule. To some extent, the computer centralizes the scheduling process. If mathematical models are properly used, the computer can produce high-quality schedules. The system will also facilitate the incorporation of standard personnel policies into the schedule, and the policies can be applied uniformly over all nursing units. It will also add more stability to the entire nursing department. The advantages of computerized scheduling are most dramatically apparent in situations where nurses rotate frequently among shifts and where nursing environments are subject to chronic change. Computer-aided, centralized schedules minimize the time spent on preparing and maintaining schedules.

NEW NURSING SPECIALTIES

Management should clearly understand the definitions of registered nurses, licensed practical nurses, and nurse aides, as well as other ancillary nurse personnel jobs, if it is going to understand properly the staffing standards to different nursing modalities (and to evaluate nurse scheduling methods). History provides an understanding of the classic nursing roles of the head nurse, general duty or staff nurse, and the nurse aide. The newer categories of nursing specialists require some additional definition.[11] These definitions could be particularly beneficial to the financial managers who see job or position descriptions written into the budget. The financial manager should understand where this "new breed" position fits into the complete nursing budget equation. The nursing service may in fact have added many new nursing specialists onto their position control budget.

There are four new positions that have evolved or have become more popular over the last decade and that may have an impact on the hospital's budget as well as its nurse staffing and scheduling. These are the clinical nurse specialists, the nurse clinicians, the nurse practitioners, and the nurse midwives.

Clinical Nurse Specialists

Clinical nurse specialists have master's degrees in a specialized clinical discipline such as pediatrics, obstetrics, or psychiatry. Nationwide, there seems to be a trend toward certifying clinical nurse specialists. One of the objectives in creating this new specialty is to return the nurse to the patient's bedside and to have a greater impact on direct patient care. Also, it is hoped that the clinical nurse specialists will provide greater comprehensiveness, continuity, and coordination of patient services by functioning as partners with the physician rather than as handmaidens or in other subservient roles.

Nurse Clinicians

Nurse clinicians are nurses in the middle-level position of nursing organization and nursing practice. Nurse clinicians have demonstrated advanced clinical competence and may provide clinical leadership for the nursing personnel working on the unit. They generally function as patient care leaders. They may be prepared at any RN level in nursing service; they may have a diploma, a bachelor's degree, or a master's degree,

Nurse Practitioners

Nurse practitioners function primarily in the ambulatory care setting. They may be graduates of any level of nursing program. Following graduation, a 4- to

12-month apprenticeship (or further study) in a formal program is required in order to become a practitioner. Nurse practitioners are most common in obstetrics, family practice, and pediatrics. In many cases, they work closely with physicians in rendering outpatient care. In fact, in some instances they have "hung out their own shingles." Frequently, nurse practitioners will function in areas that overlap the traditional doctor outpatient roles. They may take medical histories, do physical assessments on patients, and do patient medical screening.

Nurse Midwives

Since the introduction of the nurse midwife in the United States in the rural areas of Kentucky, the concept and the use of midwives has grown. A certified midwife (CMW) is a registered nurse who has received advanced training in two disciplines, nursing and midwifery.[12] Nurse midwives may be certified by the American College of Nurse Midwives. They attend healthy women during their prenatal, labor, delivery, and postpartum phases. They also are involved in certain aspects of the newborn, family planning, and routine gynecological care. Nurse midwives work as an integral part of the team concept of obstetrics and are dependent on physician consultation and referral in case of patient complications.

NURSING COST EFFECTIVENESS

Nursing may be the most important department in fulfilling the hospital's objective of patient care. The nurses constitute the hospital's single largest group of employees. Because the nursing service department represents a major portion of the hospital's expense budget, nurses will come under increasingly stringent cost controls in the future, both from within the hospital and from sources outside the hospital. Students of hospital management, nursing students, and physicians should be knowledgeable about nursing, its definitions, and its problems if they are going to be cost effective agents for their hospitals.

SPECIAL CARE UNITS

Special care units have developed with today's increased technology and modern medical advances. Over the last decade, special care units have multiplied and matured. The sophisticated modern hospital may have a variety of special care facilities to manage and to maintain patients with special illnesses and injuries. These facilities may include intensive care units for medicine and surgery, special cardiac care units, hemodialysis or renal dialysis centers, inpatient psychiatric units, inpatient alcoholic and drug addiction units, and skilled nursing facilities for long-term care. A special unit need not be based in the hospital; it may be constituted as a hospital home care program. Home care involves professionals (nurses and physicians) who attend patients in their homes. Inpatient pediatric units are not considered as special care units, since the cases are generally integrated into medical/surgical nursing principles and are very common in hospitals. Almost 50 percent of the hospitals that support the American Hospital Association have pediatric units.

Intensive Care Units

The best-established type of special care unit in the hospital is the intensive care unit (ICU). Over 60 percent of all hospitals in the country have ICUs. There are 3,880 such units in the hospital systems of the country.[13] ICU units were established to meet clinical demands of the hospitalized patients and their physicians. Their purpose is to manage the critically ill patient who is in a precarious clinical status and requires "eagle eye" supervision. The ICUs handle both surgical and medical cases. ICU cases could be patients in shock, stroke victims, or persons with heart failures, serious infections, respiratory distress, and so forth. The establishment of separate ICU units in hospitals was a major step forward in modern hospital care. By marshalling the hospital's resources in one geographical area, it is much easier and efficient to provide high quality care. Not only are sophisticated equipment and instrumentation available in ICUs, but a highly concentrated nursing staff is also used. These nursing personnel have to be particularly well prepared in a wide variety of postoperative cases as well as medical cases.

A special offshoot of the ICUs is the neonatal intensive care unit that specializes in the management of critical health problems in the newborn. Caring for the critically ill newborn requires a specially trained nurse and physician. The neonatal intensive care units have had great success in the handling of premature infants, giving them a new lease on life. According to one physician, "these units have changed the survival statistics dramatically."[14]

Coronary Care Units

The ICUs in hospitals gave birth to Coronary Care Units or CCUs. CCUs may be quite familiar to the ordinary consumer of health care, since they have grown in popularity over the past ten years. A review of the status of CCUs shows that in 1968 there were few such units in the country. Today, nearly all the 7,000 hospitals in America have CCU capacities. If one includes those facilities that have CCU capacities in their ICUs with the units that are only CCUs, there are over 5,600 CCUs in operation today.[15]

The CCUs do for patients what the ICUs do for severe medical and surgical patients. However, the CCU has not had the dramatic impact in saving lives as its predecessor, the ICU, has had. In fact, according to one observer,

> Some authorities on health care costs are currently questioning the need for a unit in every hospital. They point to the data and claim the small reduction in heart attack deaths is not worth the resources. The main problem in saving individuals stricken by heart attacks is that the majority who are going to die do so before they reach the hospital. This is why many large cities have developed sophisticated paramedic transport teams. As an adjunct to the CCU, these teams are adding an extra measure of success to coronary care medicine.[16]

For both ICUs and CCUs, it is usual to have a medical director assigned either full-time, part-time, or rotating to manage medically the units. Individual attending physicians manage their own patients. However, because there is a medical director, the attending physicians have to relinquish some of the old concept of total and complete control over their patients and realize that their care is a shared responsibility in these two intensive care units.

The nurse's role in these units is critical. The nurses should be intelligent observers, and they must be able to interpret changes in a patient. Under critical circumstances, they might have to diagnose and even treat the patient. One of the prime objectives of the CCU is to detect early signs of impending cardiac disaster so that it can be treated before cardiac arrest takes place.

Patient Monitoring Equipment

Along with the meteoric rise of the ICUs and CCUs, a spectacular development in patient care has been in the use of electronic monitoring equipment. The selection of this equipment should be based on high selectivity and detailed planning. Extensive use of monitoring equipment does not reduce the number of nursing personnel required to care for patients. There is still no substitute for the personal care of a nurse.

The monitoring equipment may vary from hospital to hospital depending on the complexity of the unit, the needs of the patients, and the resources of the hospital. The equipment can be used for routine evaluation of blood pressure, pulse, respiration, temperature, and other selected physical and physiological conditions. It is important to have built-in alarm systems that will warn the staff of critical changes in the patient's condition. Specific suggestions for cardiac monitoring equipment include oscilloscopes at the patient's bedside supplemented by heart rate meters with audio and visual alarms, pacemakers with automatic or manual controls, and integral lead selectors for obtaining complete ECG recordings. At the nurses' station, there is generally a central panel that includes oscilloscope and heart rate meters with audio and visual alarms.

Nonacute Special Care Units

There are a variety of special care units that are not geared for life-threatening situations. One of the best examples is the renal dialysis centers that have been increasing in number over the last decade. The American Hospital Association reports that there are 1,043 inpatient dialysis units and an additional 715 outpatient units in this country. The renal dialysis centers provide artificial kidney support for patients whose kidneys have stopped functioning properly. These units, unlike the CCUs and ICUs, provide long-term care needs for patients. They accommodate outpatients. Because of the medical advances in the surgical transportation of kidneys and the medical treatment of dialysis patients, many suffering from this ailment have a chance for a productive life today.

An increasing number of hospitals are also turning to inpatient psychiatric units as specialty care areas. A recent report showed that 1,203 or 19 percent of the country's general hospitals have inpatient psychiatric units.[17] If one adds these to the 465 inpatient alcoholic and drug-related units, one can see that these two areas of medicine are starting to grow in the inpatient hospital environment.

Long-Term Care Facilities

For the hospitalized patient who is unable to return to home, hospitals have become involved in reaching out into the community with home care programs. Presently, there are only a few home care programs in this country sponsored by hospitals—482 at last count. However, with the continued push toward cost containment, there seems to be great promise for more home care programs. More hospitals have become involved in long-term or nursing-home beds within their facilities; 852 or 13.5 percent of all hospitals have skilled nursing facilities. The patients in these facilities are generally recovering from strokes, severe orthopedic accidents, or a severe medical illness. There are two kinds of nursing homes: (1) skilled nursing facilities (SNFs), and (2) lower-level nursing facilities called intermediate care facilities (ICFs).

NOTES

1a. American Hospital Association, *Hospital Administrative Services,* 1979.

1b. Hospital Indicators, "A Summary of Trends in Hospital Employment," *Hospitals, JAHA,* September 16, 1980, p. 65.

2. Joseph K. Owen, *Modern Concepts of Hospital Administration* (Philadelphia, Pa.: W.B. Saunders Co., 1962), p. 510.

3. Ibid.

4. John McGiboney, *Principles of Hospital Administration* (New York, N.Y.: G.P. Putnam's Sons, 1969), p. 435.

5. McGiboney, *Principles,* p. 436.

6. Rockwell Schulz and Alton C. Johnson, *Management of Hospitals* (New York, N.Y.: McGraw-Hill Book Co., 1976), p. 92.

7. U.S. Department of the Army, *Staffing Guide for U.S. Army Hospitals,* DA—Pamphlet 20-577.

8. D. Michael Warner, "Nurse Staffing, Scheduling, and Relocation in the Hospital," *Hospital and Health Services Administration,* Summer 1976, pp. 77-90.

9. Phyllis Giovannetti, "Understanding Patients' Classification Systems," *Journal of Nursing Administration,* February 1979, p. 4.

10. Warner, "Nurse Staffing," pp. 84-85.

11. Schulz and Johnson, *Management of Hospitals.*

12. Eunice K.M. Ernst, "The Evolving Practice of Midwifery," *Health Law Project Library Bulletin,* September 1979, p. 290.

13. American Hospital Association, *Hospital Statistics* (Chicago, Ill.: AHA, 1979), p. 192.

14. Ibid., p. 169.

15. Ibid.

16. Ronald Gotz and Arthur Kaufman, *The People's Hospital Book* (New York, N.Y.: Crown Publishers, Inc., 1978), p. 168.

17. American Hospital Association, *Hospital Statistics,* p. 196.

Part V

Tests and Results

Chapter 11

Key Ancillary Services

Ancillary ∿ Surgical specimens ∿ Pathologist ∿Registered medical technologist ∿ Nuclear Medicine ∿ William Roentgen ∿ Radiologic technologist ∿ Radiologist ∿ Nurse anesthetist ∿ Informed consent for surgery ∿ Anesthesiologist

INTRODUCTION

The hospital's ancillary departments may also be called professional service departments. Literally, ancillary means a department that assists the physician in diagnosis or in the treatment of the patient. Ancillary is defined as a cost (having expenses) and revenue center (able to bill the patient for services) within the hospital which requires, either by regulation or third party urging, either that a physician direct the department or that a physician provide guidance and supervision over the department. In other words, what differentiates an ancillary service department from other hospital departments is that it is able to charge the patient directly, thereby generating revenue for the hospital, and it must be under the direction of a physician.

Ancillary departments are very complex because their charge structure is different and consists of many individual tests. In addition, the departments have highly sophisticated equipment and a variety of well-trained technical staff. Another factor that makes these departments complex for management is physician compensation. There are a variety of ways in which the physicians who direct these departments may be reimbursed.

A typical large community hospital will have the following ancillary departments: clinical laboratory, radiology (x-ray), physical therapy, inhalation therapy, anesthesiology, EKG (electrocardiography, heart station), and EEG (electroencephalography). To illustrate the function of the organization and how ancillary departments relate to the physicians and to the patients, the following sections provide some details and an analysis of three major ancillary departments: clinical laboratories, radiology, and anesthesiology.

CLINICAL LABORATORIES DEPARTMENT

Clinical laboratories, another term for pathology departments, are of rather recent origin. Yet, in their relatively short period of existence, they have undergone tremendous growth. Just before World War I, a typical pathology department in a hospital was small and ill-equipped. Pathologists spent most of their time doing simple urinalyses, blood counts, and a few chemical determinations in bacteriology. Only a few surgical specimens (tissue removed by the physician during surgery) were examined, and only a few autopsies were performed. After World War I, the pathology and clinical laboratory departments began to grow. Physicians, having learned the value of pathology services from their war experiences, began to demand such services in civilian hospitals. At the same time, as discoveries and advances became more widely adopted in a very short period of time, the number of medical journals began to increase.

Between 1875 and 1900, bacteriology reached its golden age. In fact, most of the important pathogenic microorganisms were isolated in this period. However, it was several years before these techniques became widely applied. It was not until 1937 that blood banking was used as a practical procedure in hospitals. Blood banking as a regular service in hospitals is concerned with such blood procedures as cross-matching, compatibility testing, and the preparation and storage of blood prior to transfusion. Following World War II, additional growth occurred. New knowledge on how to expose health and disease problems proliferated. Diagnostic radioisotopes, exfoliative cytology, molecular diseases, practical virology, and fluorescent studies were introduced. Today, the architect who designs a new pathology department faces quite a problem in attempting to guess what new frontiers of pathology will be established.

Functions

A hospital's clinical laboratory has a number of functions, but its primary purpose is to provide information to assist physicians and other members of the health team in the diagnosis, prevention, and treatment of disease. This primary mission is accomplished by performing tests in the laboratory. Related functions of the clinical laboratory depend on the size and complexity of the hospital; these can involve training programs and research.

One of the important ways a laboratory improves the quality of medicine is through its formal reports, especially on post-mortem examinations and on examinations of tissues removed in surgical operations (surgical specimens). Tissue committees serve as a classic quality control mechanism whereby practicing surgeons can measure and improve their clinical performance in the hospital.

Organization

The department is organized under the leadership and directorship of a pathologist. This is a licensed physician who specializes in the practice of pathology and is usually eligible for certification or certified by the American Board of Pathology in either clinical or anatomical pathology, or perhaps both.

The department itself can be divided into two major sections, a clinical pathology division and an anatomical pathology section. The clinical laboratory and pathology services fall into two areas: (1) those performed directly by the pathologist and (2) those performed under the pathologist's responsibility and supervision but actually conducted by a medical technologist.

It is the pathologist's role to examine all surgical specimens (including autopsies, frozen sections, and tissue consultations). Under the pathologist's supervision, a medical technologist's functions fall into these areas: (1) bacteriology, (2) biochemistry, (3) blood bank, (4) hematology, (5) tissue preparation, (6) organ banks which certain hospitals have to store human organs and tissues used in transplant surgery (for example, corneas and kidneys), and (7) nuclear medicine and isotopes. In some hospitals, nuclear medicine may come under the radiology department. Nuclear medicine, like x-ray, is a valuable technique in diagnosis and in treatment. Diagnostically, it is used widely in studies of the brain, liver, and lungs. In addition, it is used to detect problems of the bone, kidney, and thyroid. Recently it has been used a great deal for evaluating cardiovascular functions.

Staffing

The majority of employees in the pathology department are registered medical technologists or medical laboratory technicians. A registered technologist must complete a bachelor's degree in an accredited college or university studying specified science courses in a school of medical technology approved by the Council on Medical Education and the Hospitals of the American Medical Association. The technologist must then pass an examination given by the Board of Registry of Medical Technologists.

There may be some non-registered personnel working in the clinical laboratory, since there is a shortage of qualified personnel in certain parts of the country. From time to time, persons with Ph.D. degrees in special science disciplines (such as chemistry) work in the department. Medical technology is a growing field and is becoming more standardized as years go on. Many of the medical technologists are comparatively young women; there are not many men in the field.

The number of employees will vary with the workload in the department. Departments that are heavily involved in teaching or research or that handle outside requests will obviously vary in staffing patterns. A specific hospital staffing pattern can only be determined after an on-site analysis is conducted and knowledge of the specific workloads within the hospital is available.

As for the medical technologists themselves, there have been studies that suggest what the average workload for a technologist should be per year. These studies consider the types of tests and indicate the differences between hospitals that have a high, medium, or low volume. A staffing and workload analysis is critical when one determines how much space and equipment is needed to run a proper laboratory operation. Government studies show that most hospital laboratories have been showing annual workload increases of approximately 10 percent, which indicates that the workload will be doubled in approximately nine years. This explosion of testing has caused severe expansion problems for hospital laboratories. However, experience with improved techniques in automation suggests that a greater volume of work can be done in the same work area, depending on the clinical laboratory involved.[1]

Location and Physical Facilities

Laboratory facilities are usually found either in the basement or on the first floor. If they are on the first floor, they are more accessible to the outpatients who are sent to the laboratory. It is not as important for inpatients to come to this area, since much of the laboratory's work (that is, collecting specimens) is done on the nursing units.

In determining the overall size of the laboratory, it is important that consideration be given to each functional technical unit—that is, microbiology, chemistry, hematology, and pathology. Only after the size of each individual unit has been established can architectural layouts be properly constructed to fit into the complete program of the laboratory department. The square-foot-per-patient-bed ratio is no longer considered an adequate guide for determining the size of a laboratory. Any plans for a laboratory should be based on work volumes within specific ranges within the laboratory itself. For example, 40,000 to 75,000 tests equates to so many square feet. Since most of the hospitals in this country have between 150 and 200 beds, a typical plan for such a size hospital is shown in Figure 11-1. It includes separate work units for all technical sections—hematology, urinalysis, biochemistry, histology, serology, and bacteriology. Special support areas for glass washing and sterilizing are also available. The pathologist's office and the secretarial/reception area are in a separate cubicle. These are the main elements in a community hospital's layout.

Figure 11-1 Typical 150-200 Bed Hospital Clinical Laboratory

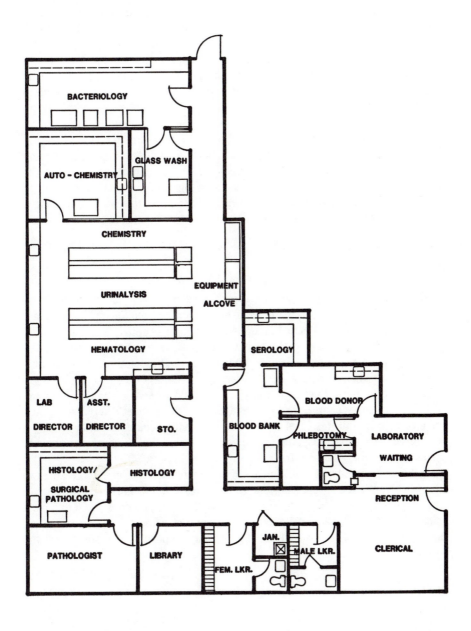

Source: Medifac, Inc., Elkins Park, Pa.

Reports and Records

The basic function of the laboratory is to provide testing to aid the physician in the diagnosis and treatment of the patient. It is essential that the test results be placed in report format and that they be promptly and accurately provided to the physicians and health professionals who need to know the results. With the 10 percent growth per year in pathology, there has also been a growth in the complexity of recordkeeping and reports. Most of these reports are handled in some manual fashion in many hospitals. Typically, tests are requested in writing on a doctor's order sheet. Then the requests are sent to the laboratory on a request form. Following the completion of the tests, the report is noted on the sheet. A copy is generally kept in the laboratory, and the original is sent back to the nursing unit for inclusion in the patient's medical record. Although this sounds simple, the massive volume in a busy hospital makes this a logistical and technical challenge for management. Recently, hospitals have been experimenting with computerized recordkeeping for laboratory reports.

Physicians' Compensation

The method of compensation to the pathologist for services rendered is very similar to the compensation arrangements for other ancillary department physicians and other hospital-based physicians. Generally, ancillary physicians are under some form of contractual arrangement with the hospital. There are a wide variety of contractual arrangements available to an administrator and a board of trustees when hiring a physician for the laboratory. These arrangements are also applicable to other ancillary service physicians. Common contractual arrangements include the following: the physicians could receive a percentage of the department's gross charges or a percentage of the department's net income; they might be given a professional fee-for-service; or they could be paid as hospital employees. In some hospitals the physicians lease the ancillary department, managing it somewhat as a franchise.

It should be noted that, unlike many of the other physicians who serve patients, these hospital-based specialists work under special contracts. These specialists—radiologists, anesthesiologists, and pathologists—could be considered to have a monopoly within the hospital, since, once they sign a contract, other competing specialists in their discipline outside of their group are not allowed to practice in the hospital.

Summary

The hospital clinical laboratory has become an essential element in the care of the patient within the hospital. Laboratory tests and examinations are growing rapidly in numbers and complexity. Since diagnosis and research in medical care are also extremely broad and intensive, the hospital pathologist becomes a critical element in the care of the patient. On the other hand, much of the testing in the laboratory is of routine nature and has been relegated to sophisticated equipment that can produce numerous tests in a brief period of time.

The pathologist is the spokesman not only for the ancillary department, but in a way is the conscience of the medical staff. The pathologist's crucial role on the tissue committee involves interpreting and guiding physicians' practices through laboratory procedures and tests. Thus this department and the pathologist in particular are key elements in the hospital's quality assurance program.

RADIOLOGY DEPARTMENT

If diagnosis is the cornerstone of modern medical medicine, then the radiology department is the cornerstone of medical diagnosis. The field of radiology had its beginning on November 8, 1895, when an astute observer and professor of physics at the University of Wurzburg in Bavaria, Wilhelm Roentgen, discovered x-rays. The discovery traveled quickly. Within a matter of weeks, physicists and physicians throughout the world were producing x-rays of various types. They were quickly applied to the practice of medicine.

X-rays, when properly applied, permit a trained physician to recognize many medical conditions not otherwise diagnosable in a living patient. In addition, radiation beams, carefully administered in sufficient doses have been found to be an effective treatment method for many diseases. These beams, emitted from x-ray tubes, gave birth to such devices as datatrons and cyclatrons, which are so important in therapeutic radiology. Today considerable progress is being made toward further use of diagnostic and therapeutic radiation procedures.

Functions

The principal functions of the radiology (x-ray) department are to assist the physicians and other health team members in the diagnosis and therapy of a patient's disease through the use of radiography, fluoroscopy, and radioisotopes. High energy machines such as linear accelerators, employing high particle acceleration, are also used in radiotherapy. There are several special procedures or diagnostic methods used in a modern hospital x-ray department. Fluoroscopy is a means by which body structures are viewed by sending x-rays through the body part to be examined and then observing the shadows cast on a fluorescent (glowing) screen. Cineradiography is a means of converting the fluorescent screen images into radiographs or even into motion pictures. Stereoscopy is the method of taking two radiographs from slightly different angles, thereby allowing physicians to view the body structure in three dimensions. There is also a commonly used procedure called angiography, which is the technique of using a contrast medium and injecting it into the patient's blood vessel, thereby allowing the blood supply (with the contrast medium) to reveal the structure and state of health of the organ.

Today, there is a newer x-ray method in common use. It is called computerized tomography (CT). In the CT method, a carriage is rotated, allowing an x-ray team to scan a narrow cross section of the body. Many such scans are taken—perhaps as many as 180—at very small distances from each other. These images are then collected and displayed with the use of a computer. In the average community hospital, 90 percent of the workload in the x-ray department consists of radiography (making a record on x-ray film by means of radioactivity) and fluoroscopy (x-ray examinations of deep structures by means of roentgen rays using a fluorescent screen).

A secondary mission of the radiology department is to engage in essential research for medical advancement and to participate in educational programs for hospital residents and in inservice programs for the medical staff. Finally, the hospital might be involved in the training of radiologic technologists and other x-ray technical specialists.

Organization

In large hospitals, the radiology department may be organized into three separate sections: diagnostic radiology, therapeutic radiology, and nuclear medicine. In small hospitals, these may be arranged in one organization. The department is under the general direction and supervision of a competent radiologist, a graduate of a medical school who is licensed to practice in the state. This person is appointed as a member of the medical staff and should have considerable specialized training in radiology, either diagnostic or therapeutic or both, and be certified by the American Board of Radiology. Frequently, the radiologist supervises a person called the chief x-ray technician. The radiologist is the clinical department head and accordingly has all the medical-administrative responsibilities. In the larger context, the radiologist, as administrator of the department, is responsible to the administrator of the hospital; as a specialist concerned with the quality of care, the radiologist is responsible to the medical staff. Members of the medical staff send their patients to the department for diagnosis and treatment. The outpatient department sends approximately 50 percent of all the x-ray work, including that from the emergency department. The various inpatient nursing units also send patients down from the unit during the working day.

Location and Physical Facilities

The x-ray department should be located on the first floor of the hospital and should be conveniently accessible to both outpatients and inpatients. If possible, it is preferable to locate the x-ray department close to elevators and adjoining the outpatient department. It is best to locate the department in a wing of the hospital with the x-ray rooms at the extreme end of the wing. In such a configuration, the traffic pattern through the department will be minimized, and less shielding from the x-rays will be required due to the exterior walls around the x-ray rooms.

A well-planned, x-ray diagnostic department will ensure an efficient flow of service, allowing patients to be scheduled properly and expediently with a minimum of movement and distance for both the x-ray staff and the patients. The number of x-ray machines to be installed in the unit will depend, of course, on the size of the hospital, the number of beds in the hospital, and the community that the hospital serves.

Flexibility in the design of the department is important, particularly in a smaller hospital. It is a prerequisite for the handling of a potential increase in the workload and volume. If sufficient space is allocated to begin with, an increase in volume can be handled quite easily by adding additional staff members and installing another machine. When designing and planning a radiology department, or reviewing whether a radiology department should be expanded, diagnostic radiology standards for room utilization are extremely helpful. There may be individual variations due to the complexity of the examination mix; however, there are guidelines that can be used in determining the number of examination rooms necessary in the x-ray suite. One figure shows that approximately 6,000 examinations per room per year is average.[2] A typical layout for a diagnostic x-ray suite for a 150 to 200 bed hospital is shown in Figure 11-2.

Staffing

The basic employee in the radiology department is the radiologic technologist or x-ray technician. There must be a sufficient number of these employees in the department to respond to the patients' needs. These technologists should be trained in x-ray work and should be eligible for membership in the American Society of Radiologic Technologists. Technicians perform their work under the supervision of the radiologist and usually a chief technician. It is estimated that one certified radiologist is needed for every 25 revenue patients per day.[3] The number of technicians required for this workload may vary between two and three. Factors to be considered are the patients' status (whether or not they are ambulatory) and whether the technicians transport the patients themselves.

Figure 11-2 Typical 150 to 200 Bed Hospital Diagnostic X-ray Suite

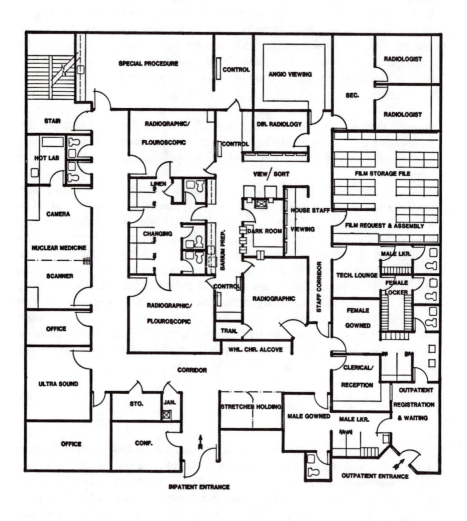

Source: Medifac, Inc., Elkins Park, Pa.

DEPARTMENT OF ANESTHESIA

The development of anesthesia began with the introduction of ether by Dr. Morton in 1847. Unlike the development of anesthesia in Great Britain, the practice of anesthesia in the United States was not always a strictly medical discipline. Though there were some surgeons who became interested in the problems of anesthesia, these represented only a minority. It was not until the 1930s when the study of the physiology of trauma in surgery began to unfold that physicians became acutely interested in the discipline of anesthesiology. Prior to that time, nurse anesthetists were involved in the giving of anesthesia. The Association of Nurse Anesthetists was formed in 1931. Since that time, the association has been a significant force in improving the standards for the training and education of nurse anesthetists. Anesthesia received a great boost during World War II, when many of the physicians in the military, particularly in the army, were given training in anesthesia before being sent to the hospitals to work.

There has been a dramatic growth in the discipline of anesthesia. In 1940, there were approximately 38 hospitals offering residency programs in anesthesiology.[4] In the same year, there were only 105 board-certified anesthesiologists. Today, there are approximately 675 residency programs and over 13,000 board-certified anesthesiologists in the United States.[5]

Functions

The anesthesia department has three main functions: (1) to render a patient insensible to pain during a surgical procedure, (2) to control the patient's physiology during the procedure and to follow the patient during the immediate postoperative period, and (3) to manage and supervise the therapy by inhalation of gaseous substances. The anesthesia department is also responsible for providing local or block anesthesia in certain surgical procedures and diseases.

Hospital administrators, nurses, physicians, and anesthesiologists all must be aware that patients going to surgery have to sign certain permission slips (informed consent for surgery) prior to surgery. A patient must be informed about the surgical procedure and the liabilities and risks involved before signing the permit to undergo the procedure.

Organization

Most hospitals have a separate department of anesthesiology. Those hospitals that do not have a separate department usually include anesthesia as a function of the department of surgery. Most often, the department of anesthesiology is headed by a physician who is trained in the medical discipline of anesthesia and, hopefully, is board certified. The department may have more than one physician anesthesiologist. It is quite common to have nurse anesthetists, that is, registered nurses who have completed a formalized post-RN anesthesia program or school. Both the physician specialist and the nurse anesthetist administer anesthesia. When a physician anesthesiologist is not available, hospitals use nurse anesthetists exclusively to administer anesthesia. The responsibility for this department is then delegated to either the chief of surgery or to another designated person. In such cases, the operating surgeon is responsible for the professional acts of the nurse anesthetists.

Staffing

The precise number of physician anesthetists and nurse anesthetists employed in a given hospital will depend upon the number and types of surgical procedures and the number of obstetrical deliveries in the hospital. Personnel in the anesthesia department are required to be on call; this, of course, has an impact on staffing patterns. The nurse anesthetists, depending on the contractual arrangement between the anesthesiologist and the hospital, either work directly for the anesthesiologist or are hospital employees. In any event, the nurse anesthetists function under the technical supervision of the anesthesiologist.

NOTES

1. U.S. Department of Health, Education, and Welfare, Public Health Service, Division of Hospitals and Medical Facilities, *Planning the Laboratory for the General Hospital*, p. 30.
2. Hospital Survey Committee, *Utilization of Facilities for Diagnostic Radiology* (Philadelphia, Pa.: Hospital Survey Committee, 1975), p. 9.
3. Joseph K. Owen, *Modern Concepts of Hospital Administration* (Philadelphia, Pa.: W.B. Saunders Co., 1962), p. 308.
4. Ibid., p. 320.
5. American Medical Association, *Physician Distribution and Medical Licensure in the U.S.* (Chicago, Ill.: 1967).

Chapter 12

Other Ancillary Services

Key Terms

Pulmonary function studies ∼ Cardiologist ∼ Stress testing ∼ Physical therapist ∼ Occupational therapist ∼ Speech therapist ∼ Fee-for-service ∼ Formulary ∼ Markup purchase ∼ Red book and blue book ∼ Floor stock ∼ Patient chargeable items ∼ Unit dose ∼ Harrison Narcotic Law ∼ Detail man

RESPIRATORY CARE DEPARTMENT

A discipline closely related to anesthesiology is respiratory therapy. The respiratory care field has developed rapidly under the sponsorship of such organizations as the American College of Physicians and the American Society of Anesthesiologists. In today's hospital, respiratory therapy is an extremely important facet of the diagnosis and treatment of certain categories of patients. The Respiratory Care Department at one time was known as the inhalation therapy department. The older term referred to the treatment of patients with the use of oxygen and other agents. The Respiratory Care Department embodies the therapeutic value of oxygen and other agents together with, among the newer studies and techniques, pulmonary function studies and blood gas analysis. The department is particularly important in the treatment and diagnosis of patients with pulmonary disease and certain cardiac ailments. The Respiratory Care Department continues to grow, not only in scope of responsibility, but also as a cost and revenue center for the hospital. It has become, in many institutions, a major ancillary department.

The JCAH has indicated that the "medical direction of the Respiratory Care Department shall be provided by a physician member of the active staff, who has a special interest in the knowledge, diagnosis, treatment, and assessment of respiratory problems. Whenever possible, this physician should be qualified by special training and/or experience in the management of acute and chronic respiratory problems."[1] The commission stipulates that respiratory care services "shall be

111

supervised by a technical director, who is registered or certified by the National Board for Respiratory Therapy, Inc. or has the documented equivalent education, training and/or experience."[2]

The respiratory therapy department is involved in both diagnostic and therapeutic treatment of inpatients and outpatients. All procedures given to the patients are performed either by the physician or by the trained respiratory therapist. These procedures can be administered to the patient only upon the prescribed written orders of a physician.

ELECTROENCEPHALOGRAPHY

One of the more specialized ancillary services in hospitals is the electroencephalography or EEG testing service. This is generally part of the neurosurgery or neurology section of the hospital or medical staff. This service is an indispensible tool for solving neurosurgical or neurological problems. The EEG test measures the electrical brain activity of the patient. It is frequently used when patients have suffered serious head injuries; in such circumstances, an EEG test can be a lifesaver. EEG testing was formerly used primarily for the diagnosis of seizures and the detection of tumors. However, in recent years the EEG test has been utilized in analyzing many problems, from fainting and mild headaches to epileptic disorders and severe trauma from a head injury. The test is conducted by highly trained technicians upon a physician's order. The EEG test has to be conducted in a room where extraneous noise cannot be picked up. If the room is not perfectly situated, certain artifacts will appear on the EEG readout and make it worthless. The EEG laboratory does not have a high volume, like laboratory and x-ray. Frequently, however, EEG lab technicians are on 24-hour call for emergency determinations. EEG tests are used in determining both the first signs of life and the last signs of life coming from the brain. Often the EEG test can be the means of determining whether the patient is legally alive or dead.

There are hybrids of the EEG technique that include studies when the patient is asleep or partially asleep. The sleep EEGs are particularly important in the study of different types of epilepsy. With the advent of CAT Scanners, some people believe that EEGs have lost some of their value. However, the EEG printouts continue to be used; rather than the brain scan replacing this ancillary study, the EEG test is frequently used in combination with the brain scan.

ELECTROCARDIOGRAPHY

Throughout the years, the diagnostic tool of electrocardiography (EKG) has proven to be a necessity in the general community hospital. The EKG is used most frequently on patients having cardiac disease, suspected cardiac disease, or complications of cardiac disease. It is also useful as a chest baseline test prior to surgery. If an electrocardiogram is abnormal, detailed information regarding the diagnosis and management of the patient is provided; this makes the course of the patient's treatment much more reasonable and scientific. An electrocardiogram is taken with special equipment to produce an electrocardiograph. The basic EKG machine is a table-type of apparatus on wheels that is rolled to the inpatient's bedside. It is operated by highly skilled technicians.

The interpreter of the cardiogram is usually a cardiologist or an internist who is skilled in reading electrocardiogram tracings. The technician must be trained to take multilead tracings, that is, tracings from the twelve leads that are normally attached to the patient to obtain a standard electrocardiogram.

Financial Arrangements

The cardiologist or interpreter is usually paid for each electrocardiogram interpreted; however, the payment could be in the form of a fixed salary. The financial arrangements are not usually as complex as those with the radiologist, pathologist, and anesthesiologist.

Physical Facilities

The electrocardiograph service is usually a mobile service, in that the technicians frequently must go to the patients' beds while they are inpatients and take tracings while the patients are resting. However, for outpatients and occasional inpatients who can travel to the central cardiograph area, the service is usually located within the department of cardiology. In the department, a small room with a bed in a quiet location is the only facility necessary to conduct the electrocardiographic testing. All electrocardiograph tests are considered diagnostic procedures and must be ordered by a physician.

Different Modalities of Testing

Though the basic electrocardiogram is the most common service in hospitals, there are variations of electrocardiograph tracings that are done for different purposes to determine the special diagnostic problem. For example, stress testing is a procedure in which a patient is placed under severe stress, and the patient's heart impulses are then interpreted in those conditions. There is also echoencephalography and Holter monitoring, procedures in which a patient wears a tracing device while active for a period of hours; tracings are then made and interpreted usually through a computer reading.

EKG Systems As Shared Services

Hospitals may use a three-channel EKG cart with computerized printout attachments as part of their equipment. In this arrangement, the technician goes to the patient's bedside with an electrocardiograph cart that has a telephone receiver attached. The tracings are sent over the telephone lines to be read. The reading is then relayed to a computer that interprets the reading and prints out at the patient's bedside within 20 to 50 seconds what is called an "unconfirmed" electrocardiograph reading. It is unconfirmed because the computer has read it, not a cardiologist. The unconfirmed reading is usually confirmed by having a hospital cardiologist "overread" the computerized interpretation printout. The physician who reads the printout signs it as if the technician in the hospital had taken the tracing. The advantages of the shared computerized electrocardiogram system are basically two: (1) it provides a high degree of consistency and quality, and (2) it provides fast feedback time on the readings.

PHYSICAL MEDICINE AND REHABILITATION

The discipline of physical medicine and rehabilitation is a medical specialty concerned with the diagnosis and treatment of certain musculoskeletal defects and neuromuscular diseases and problems. Physical medicine began to emerge during World War I when the Army was involved in vocational guidance and training programs for the disabled. However, it was not until some time following World War II that the specialty became well known and formal training programs became more available.

The first three-year residency in physical medicine and rehabilitation was established at the Mayo Clinic. Today, there are only a limited number of hospitals specializing in complete physical medicine and rehabilitation services. However, it is quite common for a community hospital to have a physical therapy section supporting the medical rehabilitation programs of certain patients.

Some of the areas of rehabilitative medicine that community hospitals typically are involved in include physical therapy, occupational therapy, and speech therapy. Physical therapy is commonly prescribed by physicians, and the referred patient is evaluated and treated by the physical therapist. Hospitals may offer occupational therapy services under the direction of a physician. Finally, speech therapy is becoming more common in community hospitals. This is a therapeutic discipline that uses speech therapists and physicians to correct a patient's speech defects or to reeducate the patient who may have lost the power of speech through disease, accident, or stroke.

If a hospital has a physical medicine department, it will be headed by a physician called a physiatrist whose special interests lie in physical medicine and rehabilitation. In community hospitals, according to the JCAH standards, "the responsibility for medical direction or supervision of the rehabilitation program/services shall be vested in a physician member of the medical staff, who on the basis of training, experience and interest is knowledgeable in the rehabilitation services offered. When desired this responsibility may be assigned to a medical staff committee, the chairman of which shall provide medical direction and supervision under the committee's guidance."[3]

Physical therapy is carried out by physical therapists. These professionals have earned either a bachelor's, master's or doctoral degree in physical therapy, or they have a postbaccalaureate certificate of training. By 1990, it is expected that only postbaccalaureate training programs will be accredited. The therapist may be registered through the Registry of Physical Therapy (RPT) in appropriate states or otherwise professionally licensed by the state (licensed physical therapist or LPT) where a registry is not maintained. The therapist uses light, heat, water, electricity, ultrasound, and physical and mechanical force to treat the patient's illness or pain.

The occupational therapist is involved in treating physical disability and in teaching the patient compensatory techniques to perform daily activities, frequently with the assistance of self-help aids. The occupational therapist is also involved in perceptual testing and training. The therapist is guided by the physician when creating certain educational and functional activities to help patients.

The speech therapist works with children and adults handicapped by speech and language problems with the objective of bringing them back as close as possible to normal speech functions. Often the speech therapists are involved in stressing methods to correct speech and language deficits.

PHYSICAL THERAPY

Although physical facilities will vary widely, hospitals will usually have a large room or gymnasium for physical therapy. In this area there will be sufficient space for patient cubicles, dressing rooms, toilets and showers, running water, and a great deal of physical therapy equipment. This equipment may include diathermy units, ultrasound devices, gym mats, Hubbard tanks, parallel walking bars, ultraviolet lamps, whirlpool baths, exercising steps, progressive resistance apparatus, and treatment tables.

Physical therapists work under the direction of physicians who are usually hospital employees. The financial arrangements between the physician (physiatrist) and the hospital management are usually on a simplified salaried or "fee-for-service" basis. Fee-for-services is a method whereby a physician bills the patient or third party for each physician service rendered. Reports on the patient's therapy are recorded and made part of the patient's medical record.

THE PHARMACY

The hospital pharmacy has the role of manufacturing, compounding, and dispensing drugs and other diagnostic and therapeutic chemical substances that may be used in the hospital. Smaller hospitals may not have a regular pharmacy department; they may purchase items from a local pharmacist and maintain only a limited supply under lock and key. In larger hospitals, a full-time pharmacist is available, sometimes with one or two assistants. The pharmacist who heads the pharmacy department must be licensed and be able to provide a full range of pharmacy activities. Whether the pharmacy department manufactures certain solutions or drugs is a matter of hospital policy. For quality and economy reasons, most hospitals prefer to purchase the solutions already made, whether they be for injections or for intravenous administration. The precise selection of drugs that the hospital offers is generally determined by the medical staff through its pharmacy and therapeutics committee in concert with the hospital pharmacist. A listing of the drugs that are regularly available through the pharmacy is recorded in the hospital formulary; the list of drugs is usually by their generic names. The pharmacy may sell items to the general public in addition to the patients, but this practice is generally discouraged by administrators.

Pharmacy and Therapeutics Committee

The JCAH recommends that there be a committee of the medical staff called the pharmacy and therapeutics committee to oversee the medical aspects of the hospital's pharmacy activities. The commission suggests the following with respect to the responsibility of a pharmacy and therapeutics committee: "The development and surveillance of pharmacy and therapeutics policies and practices, particularly drug utilization within the hospital, shall be the responsibility of the medical staff and shall be carried out in cooperation with the pharmacist and with representatives of other disciplines as required."[4] The JCAH also stipulates that "the responsibilities of the individuals performing the pharmacy and therapeutic functions also include the development of a formulary or drug list that is reviewed" and that the responsibilities of the pharmacy and therapeutics committee include "the review of all untoward drug reactions and the evaluation and approval of all protocols concerned with the use of investigational or experimental drugs."[5]

Though the pharmacy and therapeutics committee recommends the standard drugs to be dispensed in the hospital, it is the pharmacist's responsibility in the vast majority of hospitals to select the brand or supplier of drug dispensed for all medication orders and prescriptions unless a specific notation to the contrary is made by the prescriber.

Drug Charges

Hospital pharmacies will charge based on the hospital charging policy. This usually involves the cost of the drugs plus a given percentage or a markup percentage. The markup could be as little as 25 percent or as great as 200 to 400 percent.

There are two ways of viewing costs in the pharmacy world. The retail and wholesale drug prices are outlined in documents called "red books." The Drug Topics Red Book and the American Druggist Blue Book include a variety of product reference material, including an extensive index of drugs. Both books are used as reference. Notwithstanding the purchase cost of the drug, the price markup must include all the labor and processing costs of the drug and overhead costs that are allocated under Medicare cost reimbursement rules. Therefore, it is not uncommon to find that an employee or a patient can purchase a drug at a retail pharmacy for less than the discounted price at a hospital pharmacy. Again, the overhead cost is allocated under Medicare. Of course the computed cost of the drugs is high.

Drug Distribution System

Once the hospital receives the drugs, they must be distributed. Distribution is primarily to the nursing units where inpatients receive the majority of the drugs dispensed by the pharmacy. Generally the drugs fall into one of three categories:

1. Items sent to the nursing units for floor stock inventory. These are items regularly stored in the unit and not charged to the patients directly. Examples of such nonchargeable items are rubbing compounds and antiseptics for wounds and bandages.
2. Patient-chargeable stock items kept in the nursing unit. These include disposable enemas and other disposable external preparations.
3. Common prescription drugs that are dispensed and charged only upon the receipt of a prescription by a physician. This category of prescription drugs represents the vast majority of drugs used and also represents the greatest cost in the pharmacy.

A common method of dispensing medication to patients is the unit dose system. The pharmacy either packages the medication or receives from vendors prepackaged medications in specific dosages. The latter method allows for better control and less waste of the drug; on the other hand, there is with this method the additional cost of packaging the drugs. A recent pharmaceutical survey showed a "substantial increase in the number of hospitals with a unit dose drug distribution system since 1975. Nearly half of the hospitals now have at least some of their beds on unit dose systems as compared with about 28% of the hospitals in 1975.''[6]

The unit dose system offers greater convenience to the hospital pharmacist, the nurses, and the patients. With this system, there is increased efficiency of operations, and preparation and distribution errors are reduced.

Control of Narcotics and Barbiturates

The hospital must exercise strict control over the dispensing of narcotics and barbiturates. These drugs must be kept under security both in the pharmacy and in the nursing units. Thorough and adequate records must be kept on narcotics and barbiturates. At the change of each nursing shift, a narcotics and barbiturates count is taken. Maintenance of narcotics in the hospital must be in conformance with the Harrison Drug Act and the Food, Drug, and Cosmetic Act for Barbiturates. Physicians must note their narcotic license number on the prescription when they order a narcotic. When they give a telephone order for narcotics to a nurse, they generally must place their written signature and number on the patient's medical record within 48 hours. Most hospitals have instituted a procedure by which narcotic orders must be reordered by the physician after a certain length of time. A definition of narcotic drugs is provided in the Comprehensive Drug Abuse Prevention and Control Act of 1970.

Generic versus Brand Name Drugs

The Federal government and other agencies are encouraging the use of generic drugs because the cost for the generic drug is considerably below that of brand names. A drug's generic name is the official (nonproprietary) name by which the drug is scientifically known, based on its chemical substance irrespective of the manufacturer. A drug's brand name or trade name is the registered trademark given to the drug by its manufacturer. The amount of generic drugs sold, compared to brand drugs, account for only 200 million dollars or 2.4 percent of the estimated 8.1 billion dollars in domestic prescription drug sales.[7]

The question is, Why is the allegiance to brand names so strong and why have not generics made a greater impact in the markets? According to a vice president of one of the large pharmaceutical houses in this country, "They want the service that major manufacturers provide and the dependability that comes with a proven track record."[8] A physician today must constantly face the question of who will bear the brunt if he is involved in a therapeutic misadventure.[9] To back up his theory, the vice president of the drug firm indicated that "one year after the State of Michigan passed a substitution law (ordering of generic drugs) the level of generic prescribing is still only around 8%."[10]

Selling Drugs to Hospitals

A discussion about hospital pharmacies and the sale of drugs would not be complete without mention of the drug "detail men" or pharmaceutical service representatives hired by the major drug manufacturing companies. These individuals provide a very valuable service, particularly to the physicians who order the drugs. Detail men frequently call on physicians to acquaint them with the advantages of their particular drugs and to introduce new products from their company that are on the market. These drug sales people receive superior training in the pharmaceutical sales business. One large pharmaceutical firm requires that their new salesmen undergo a nine-month certification process before they go into the field. Even though the detail men acquaint the physicians in the hospital with new drugs and try to reinforce the use of existing drugs, hospitals are now purchasing drugs more and more through group purchasing arrangements. A recent survey of hospitals shows that, on average, the incidence of group purchasing has nearly doubled since 1975. More than 70 percent of all hospitals are involved in some sort of hospital group purchasing arrangements for some of their drugs and supplies.[11]

Drug Use Review

One of the new functions of the pharmacy is to participate in drug use review programs within the hospital. For some time now, a number of experts in the hospital field have been emphasizing the importance of drug utilization review programs. They have encouraged the pharmacist to be active in developing criteria and standards for the use of drugs in hospitals. They also emphasize the need for pharmacists to have input into the drug utilization review process in the hospitals and to be active in identifying drug misuse and in proposing corrective measures. Drug utilization review projects have involved hospital inpatients, outpatients, and patients in long-term care facilities.

One of the specific tasks accomplished in drug utilization review programs is to have drug usage identified according to drug type. Statistics can be developed to indicate what percentage of patients receive certain types of drugs during hospitalization. Another function that the program looks into is drug usage according to diagnosis. Patient diagnoses can be reviewed to determine if any drugs are being used in the presence of a medical problem where there is contraindication, for example, steroids being used in the presence of a peptic ulcer. The record shows that pharmacies participating in drug utilization review programs have doubled since 1975, increasing from 25 to 50 percent.[12]

NOTES

1. Joint Commission on Accreditation of Hospitals, *Accreditation Manual for Hospitals*—1980 Edition (Chicago, Ill.: JCAH, 1979), p. 172.
2. Ibid.
3. Ibid., p. 162.
4. Ibid., p. 106.
5. Ibid., p. 107.
6. Michael H. Stolar, "National Survey of Hospital Pharmaceutical Service—1978," *American Journal of Hospital Pharmacy*, March 1979, p. 21.
7. James Snyder, "The Detail Man as Superhero," *Sales, Marketing and Management*, March 14, 1977, p. 46.
8. Ibid.
9. Ibid.
10. Ibid.
11. Stolar, "National Survey," p. 318.
12. Ibid., p. 316.

Part VI

Behind the Scenes

Chapter 13

Environmental Support Services

Key Terms

Executive housekeeper ⁓ Maids and porters ⁓ Isolation technique ⁓ Infection control ⁓ Par levels ⁓ Outside linen service ⁓ Laundry manager ⁓ Linen. marking ⁓ Preventive maintenance program ⁓ Requisition system ⁓ Contract maintenance ⁓ Safety committee ⁓ Security force ⁓ Boiler engineers

WHAT ARE SUPPORT SERVICES?

Hospital support services are defined as those hospital departments (or cost centers) that are not ancillary departments. These services do not generate patient revenue and are not under the professional direction of a physician as required by the JCAH. There are three types of support services in a hospital: the environmental services departments, the administrative service departments, and the patient-service departments. Environmental services include the traditional plant operation services, such as the housekeeping department, the laundry service, the maintenance department, the physical plant, and the engineering department. The patient-support services may have direct patient contact and include the dietary department, social services, and pharmacy. The administrative-support services are those nonpatient care departments that directly support the administrative mission of the hospital and include the purchasing, personnel, and volunteer departments.

These support services are all cost centers but do not generate patient revenue. Ordinarily these departments do not directly bill patients for services rendered. The departments are under the direction of a technical, professional, or administrative head; they are not required to be under the direction or supervision of a physician.

HOUSEKEEPING DEPARTMENT

Not too long ago, housekeeping in the hospital was the responsibility of the nursing service department. As nurses became more intensely trained, however, their professionalism became more apparent. Thus, the housekeeping department as a separate functional area was born. The department has two principal functions: to keep the hospital clean, and to control the linen supply. Keeping a hospital clean is not an easy task. Part of the problem is that a hospital is an active place, open 24 hours a day, every day of the year. Frequently the high traffic areas need special attention; if they are not cleaned properly, they can give a negative image to the entire hospital. There is more to cleaning a hospital than simply making sure that each room and floor are cleaned properly under the right standards. Cleanliness for both hospital visitors and the staff has two side effects: it creates a public relations image, and it has a psychological effect on the patients and their visitors. A clean hospital is perceived to be a well-organized and well-run hospital.

Staffing

The hospital housekeeping department is a labor intensive department. It uses modern, up-to-date equipment. The job of cleaning the patient rooms, corridors, offices, and lobbies of the hospital falls to the labor force, made up primarily of maids and porters. The administrative head of the department may be called the executive housekeeper, chief housekeeper, or director of housekeeping. The housekeeping organization is classical, in that it is based on a hierarchical principle with the chief housekeeper at the top, then one or two assistants (supervisors or forepersons), and maids and porters at the bottom.

Among the maids and porters, rank is based on a traditional division of labor derived from historical job descriptions. The maids are assigned light cleaning, dusting, and mopping of the floors. The porters usually do the heavy housekeeping and the furniture moving. By the nature of the cleaning process, there are more maids than porters. The maids are the front line of the housekeeping department and generally are assigned to divisions of sections or units in the hospital. Usually a nursing unit will have one maid assigned regularly with additional maids working in the evening shift or on weekends. The maids have an impact on patients in two ways. The results of their work (that is, a clean nursing unit or patient bedroom) have both a public relations and psychological effect. The maids' approaches, professionalism, attitudes, and personalities directly affect the patients, since they come in constant daily contact with patients while cleaning their rooms. A cheerful, well-informed, polite maid can add a great deal to the total image of the hospital.

There are two special cleaning problems. Whenever a patient is infected and has to be moved into isolation, the housekeeping department must properly disinfect the patient's room. The department interfaces directly with the infection control committee of the hospital in disinfecting a given area or room, using special bacterial solutions and certain misting or other kinds of techniques that have proven effective in disinfecting accommodations. The second special cleaning problem for the housekeeping department is vermin and rodent control. Unless the housekeeping department is alert at all times, there is the potential for pests and rodents to proliferate. The department wages continuous war against these pests. The department continually tests and evaluates disinfectants, house cleaning products, pest control devices, and other new materials and products that come on the market.

Linen Control

The hospital may wash and distribute its own linen by operating its own hospital laundry, or it may contract with a laundry service and receive its linen from an outside source. In either case, linen control generally falls to the housekeeping department. It is difficult to appreciate the vast number of laundry items that are required in a hospital. There are the obvious sheets, pillows, pillow cases, and blankets. Additionally, there are patient gowns, including gowns required in areas such as x-ray or the hospital clinics. Add to this the need for washing linens, face cloths, bath towels, face towels, and even paper towels that may be substituted in certain public restrooms. All of this linen control, distribution, and collection of soiled linen falls to the housekeeping department. Linen has enjoyed the effects of inflation and in itself has come to be a high cost item in the hospital budget.

One of the tasks in dealing with linen control is the establishment of regular operating levels or par levels. A par level is a level of linen inventory required for a specific period of time in a certain area. In a nursing unit, par levels are usually planned on either a daily or weekly basis. Linen control is most adequately done through controlling par levels on the nursing unit. An adjunct to the linen control system in some hospitals is the uniform distribution system. It sometimes falls to the housekeeping department to distribute uniforms for hospital personnel. In many hospitals, there are sewing rooms where a part-time or full-time employee repairs linen.

There are problems with linen control. New items are counted as they are purchased, but soiled linen is difficult to count and is therefore usually weighed. Linen supplies have been a favorite item of pilferage within hospitals.

HOSPITAL LAUNDRY

Without clean linen the hospital cannot operate properly. The laundry service produces the clean linen. Hospitals may have their own hospital laundry, built and operated on the hospital grounds. Or they may use a cooperative hospital laundry with a group of hospitals that have joined together to use an independent laundry. They can also use a commercial laundry. A final option is a complete outside linen service with both the linen and the laundry done by an outside retail launderer.

The nursing unit cannot be operated adequately if a safe, clean supply of linen is not assured. Though this sounds like a simple task, it is in fact the biggest problem of the laundry manager. The hospital laundry serves a large segment of the hospital. The nursing units need linen. The operating room uses a vast supply of clean linens. The delivery room and the x-ray department need gowns and drapes. The dietary department needs towels and drapes for the many medical trays it prepares. The central medical supply (central sterile supply), where so many of the hospital's sterile packs and instruments are wrapped, is a big user of linen. Given all these customers, there are certain basic factors that need to be in place if the laundry and the linen service in the hospital are to operate satisfactorily.

The department head of the laundry is called the laundry manager. The laundry manager must possess skills in dealing with people and should understand laundry equipment and the technical aspects of laundering through proper solutions and washing formulas. The exact number of personnel required to operate a hospital laundry will vary with the number of beds in the hospital. If the laundry is responsible for retrieving soiled linens, distributing the linens, and packing certain sterile instruments, the number of personnel will increase. To operate the laundry itself, the number of personnel required for a 100-175-bed hospital is 12; the number for a 200-300-bed hospital is in the range of 15.[1] The quantity of laundry needed must be determined. One standard recommended by the government is to have six complete sets of linen for each occupied bed. According to the government studies, the six sets would be used as follows: one set on the patient's bed, one set enroute to the laundry, one set being processed in the laundry, one set at the nursing unit ready to be used, and two sets in active storage for weekends or emergency use.[2]

Linen Control

One of the traditional and chronic problems facing hospitals is effective linen control. Without the proper amount of linen at the right time, patient care, employee morale, and economic hospital operations are all negatively affected. Effective control begins, as noted previously, in the housekeeping department with the proper par level. If the linen purchased is of high quality, the rate of replacement is reduced and the savings in cost can be measured. Most linens are either muslin or linen wrappers and drapes. Once the linen has reached the nursing floor, it is a good policy to secure it in locked linen closets, in locked linen carts, or in a dresser or a locked cabinet in the patient's room.

Another factor in linen control, especially in guarding against pilferage, is that the hospital linen should be properly marked. Linen marking (that is, a hospital name or symbol woven into the hand and bath towels) is a very effective means of reducing the temptation of people to take linens home with them. In the case of linens and sheets, decals can be affixed to the items. It is common for hospitals to have different colored linen throughout the hospital. For example, the operating room may use blue, maternity may use green, and medical-surgical nursing units may use white. It is unusual to find general hospitals that launder the patient's personal clothing.

Linen Distribution

There are two methods of distributing linen to the nursing units. Clean linen for the day should be on the nursing floor ready for use no later than the first shift (7:00 A.M.). The distribution itself is usually handled in a centralized fashion in which one or more large linen carts are regularly rotated around the nursing units from floor to floor. Another method of distributing linen, the decentralized way, is to provide each nursing unit with its own separate linen cart. With this method, a nursing unit may have a small supply of emergency linen on the floor, but the bulk of the linen is kept in the linen carts (usually under lock and key).

The Physical Plant

When the hospital owns and operates its own laundry, the facility may be in a separate building on the hospital grounds or in the hospital proper. In the latter case, it may be located in the lower levels, perhaps in the basement with separate entrances. A typical hospital laundry will have areas set aside for receiving and sorting soiled linen. Other functional areas of the laundry are the washing room and the clean linen processing room with its large tables for sorting, tumblers for drying, and machines for pressing the other linens. Besides the linen processing room, the laundry will have a clean linen and pack preparation room where the clean linen is put on shelves for storage or placed directly into the decentralized linen carts. Administrators and laundry managers are continually seeking improved automated equipment to save time.

The laundry department has two departments that it must service: the housekeeping department and the nursing service department. Since the laundry's principal customers are the nurses, the laundry manager should consult with the director of nurses (as well as the director of housekeeping) as that person tends to be at a key point in the delivery of the laundry.

MAINTENANCE DEPARTMENT

A department in the hospital that is often overlooked by patients and visitors is the maintenance department. This is especially true in a new, modern hospital. It is difficult to imagine that there could be much maintenance involved in repairing the equipment, the buildings, or the grounds. Yet when one looks at some of the older hospitals, the role that maintenance has in keeping the hospital operating properly becomes apparent. Hospital equipment and buildings were once relatively simple. With the increased complexity of hospital equipment, however, they have become more complex and an additional burden has been placed on the maintenance function of the hospital. There are essentially two aspects of maintenance: traditional maintenance and biomedical maintenance or engineering.

Traditional Maintenance

Functions

The traditional or primary function of the maintenance department is to maintain the buildings and machinery of the hospital. This includes the hot water and steam plant, the plumbing, the waste disposal system, the hospital's electrical power system (including the emergency power systems), the repair of hospital furniture, and the upkeep of painting and wall coverings of the interior and exterior of the hospital. Additionally, the department is responsible for the maintenance of the grounds and for proper landscaping, including snow removal. The department should be staffed with skilled individuals. Often plumbers, carpenters, cabinetmakers, electricians, and experienced painters are found among its skilled employees.

The functions of the maintenance department include the planning and scheduling of the work to be done, the supervision of the activities of the maintenance personnel, the handling of equipment problems, and the selection of quality personnel to work in the department. In addition, the maintenance director must maintain a proper inventory of supplies and equipment. All of these functions may be vastly improved if the maintenance department and the hospital have a preventive maintenance program.

Preventive Maintenance

Preventive maintenance is maintenance work done on a regular basis to keep the machinery and equipment from breaking down. However, the best preventive maintenance program will not prevent some breakdowns of equipment and material. The preventive maintenance program includes periodic inspections of the equipment, at which time the inspector should make minor adjustments to the apparatus. Recordkeeping is critical to an adequate preventive maintenance program; the purchase date of the item, major repairs on the equipment, and inspection reports all must be recorded.

Just as the preventive maintenance program is the cornerstone of successful hospital maintenance activity, a sensible requisition system for repairs and maintenance of equipment must be established. In emergency conditions (such as instances of stopped-up plumbing fixtures or electrical shortages), the requisition form could be sent in as a confirmation. Without an effective requisition system, the management of the activities of the maintenance department would be almost impossible. The requisition form should include the problem and the type of equipment; then the most economical way to repair or replace equipment can be determined. Based on an analysis of the requisition forms, the director of the maintenance department can support budgetary requests for increased supplies or personnel.

Contract maintenance is the use of outside maintenance experts to repair hospital equipment. Traditionally, this is done for large, complex pieces of equipment such as elevators. But as hospitals become more complex with esoteric clinical equipment, outside maintenance specialists are increasingly called in to supplement the regular maintenance staff. Usually the x-ray equipment is serviced by outside experts. The cost of these repairs should rightfully be included in the cost of hospital maintenance, even though they may show up as a direct expense in the department.

Parking Facilities

All hospitals have some need for parking. It usually falls to the maintenance department to operate and maintain the hospital's parking facilities. Convenient, safe, and adequate parking can be a big marketing plus for any hospital. Adequate parking facilities can also be helpful in recruiting a medical staff and employees. For hospitals in high crime areas, a well-lighted, very secure parking facility is important in order to retain qualified staff. The most acute need for parking occurs at the overlap time between the change of day shift (7:00 A.M. to 3:30 P.M.) and the evening shift (3:00 P.M. to 11:30 P.M.). With so many hospitals adding new wings and other facility additions, parking land has become more scarce, especially around urban hospitals. As a result, parking garages have become more popular. Multilevel parking garages provide considerable parking space on a relatively small parcel of land, which should be close or contiguous to the hospital. The hospital staff will not find the parking facilities acceptable if they are a long distance from the hospital.

Staff Functions

Generally, the maintenance director is in charge of security matters and the hospital safety program (including fire prevention). The safety program in most hospitals is organized under the leadership of the safety committee. Frequently, the maintenance director is either the chairperson or a key member of this committee. Much of the program's work is done through inspections and reports. If there is an incident involving a patient, a visitor, or an employee, an incident report is generated by the appropriate hospital personnel and forwarded to the insurance company that covers the hospital. The safety committee catalogs these incident reports, investigates them, and reports back to administration.

In its standards, the JCAH requires that fire drills be held at least quarterly on each shift of hospital personnel, especially in the larger urban hospitals.

Security

Security forces within the hospital are becoming quite common, particularly in urban hospitals. In earlier years, these security forces were staffed usually either by personnel under the direction of the maintenance department or by an outside private security agency. It is more common now for hospitals to have a separate security department that may be headed by a retired police officer. An effective security program is important not only to secure the hospital's building and equipment but also to give the employees the feeling that they are working in a closely supervised and safe environment. In addition, an effective security program conveys to the public the assurance that the hospital safeguards its property.

Plant Engineering

The plant engineering department has the responsibility to operate properly the hospital's power plant or boiler room section. Through this department, the hospital generates the energy necessary for many of the crucial functions of the hospital, including heat, hot water, and sterilizing. The plant engineering department is primarily concerned with the production and transmission of heat, power, and light. The hospital boiler room is under the direction of a boiler engineer. These individuals have training and experience in the safe operation and maintenance of the equipment necessary to produce the heat, steam, and electricity in the hospital. They are concerned primarily with the operation of the hospital's boilers. They may also be involved in heating and ventilating systems, air conditioning systems, water supplies, sewer systems, and standby electrical systems for the emergency generation of the steam, heat, light, and power.

Many states and cities have licensure laws that require boiler engineers to be examined by a board or a group of qualified men. In these cases, after passing qualification examinations, the boiler engineer receives an operating license. This license must be posted in the hospital's power plant as proof of the individual's qualifications. The engineering license primarily covers boiler operations, refrigeration, and the fundamentals of other activities related to the direction of steam.

The licensing examinations vary from state to state. In many areas, a licensed engineer is required by law to be on duty at the boiler plant at all times.

Energy Conservation

In days past when gasoline was 30 cents a gallon, energy was regarded as a cheap means of production and taken for granted. Recently, however, the cost of producing steam, through the use of either coal, oil, or gasoline, has become a very important cost function for the administrator to consider. Since hospitals are in operation seven days a week and use intensively large energy-pulling machines—such as sterilizing units in the operating room and central sterile supply and radiology units in the x-ray department—they have become targets of conservation for the government and local hospital councils as well as by third party payers such as Blue Cross. In fact, the federal government has sponsored legislation to provide grants and assistance to hospitals in conducting energy audits. The government has also provided grants to hospitals to improve their energy conservation posture. One very successful energy program was launched in Philadelphia under the auspices of the Greater Philadelphia Blue Cross. The record shows that, after three years of intensive audits and study, several hospitals drastically reduced their consumption of energy through basic energy conservation measures. Because energy costs have far outstripped other increased costs in hospital budgets over the last five years, energy conservation has become an important item for the hospital administrator and the financial structure of hospitals.

Biomedical Engineering

Beyond the traditional role of the hospital maintenance department, as technology has grown rapidly in the hospital area, another maintenance need has arisen. This is the need to maintain the highly technical clinical (biomedical) equipment that affects patient care and the safety of the hospital.

New technology is constantly moving into the health care arena. Some observers have noted that, "as early as 1969 it was estimated that there were 100,000 different machines being offered for hospital use by manufacturers, and between 1970 and 1975 the sale of just patient monitor equipment tripled."[3]

This new breed of clinical equipment, commonly referred to as biomedical equipment, covers the following areas: equipment used for patient diagnosis, including equipment that displays whole body potentials, measures physiological parameters, and analyzes specimens in the clinical laboratory; therapeutic treatment equipment; devices that apply radiant energy to the body; equipment for resuscitation, prosthesis, physical therapy, and surgical support; and patient-moni toring equipment (this refers to diagnostic devices for continuously indicating the patient's body parameters).

A hospital must have adequate maintenance for this biomedical equipment. Under the older system (under common law), the hospital was held liable for patent defects and for latent but checkable defects in its medical devices, but was not held liable for the latent uncheckable defects. Since 1976, however, under amendments to the Federal Food, Drug, and Cosmetic Act, a hospital may, as a distributor, be held liable for all device defects, including latent uncheckable defects.[4] In addition, the JCAH has revised its standards relating to biomedical equipment and indicated that the hospital should have an adequate well-trained staff to supervise and to maintain this equipment. Recently, medical device legislation has come to affect the whole area of biomedical equipment. The new technology has brought new problems to the hospital—among them, an additional burden of protecting the patients' safety and of protecting the hospital from potential malpractice suits.

Biomedical Technicians

Who are the maintenance men who work on this technical equipment? There are two recognized levels of technicians: the first level is that of the operation technician who has little formal training but perhaps a great deal of on-the-job training in the hospital. This level of technician sets up, checks, and operates the biomedical equipment. The second level involves a more technically oriented technician with specific biomedical equipment training. This individual is trained to construct and repair the esoteric equipment. One reporter has estimated that hospitals in the United States need from 5,000 to 8,000 clinical engineers to maintain this equipment.[5] The Association for the Advancement of Medical Instrumentation (AAMI) represents the clinical engineers and the biomedical equipment technicians. It also certifies these individuals. This organization estimates that there are only 300 to 400 clinical engineers actually employed today in the United States. From these figures one can see that there is an alarming shortage of and need for certified technicians.

Equipment Maintenance

There are four approaches the hospital can take to maintaining biomedical technical equipment:

1. It can establish its own inhouse program.
2. It can subscribe to and rely on a single commercial vendor to provide services.
3. It can participate in a shared service arrangement with other hospitals.
4. It can use a combination of vendors, manufacturers, representatives, and dealers to provide the maintenance of the equipment.

The last approach cited is an expensive one. With so many people involved, the legal liability of the hospital is increased. Also, patient care personnel in the hospital tend to spend more time doing maintenance. The purchasing department has an increased workload in recordkeeping. Finally, the JCAH requirements are not technically met under this arrangement. The use of multiple sources of services does not seem to be a prudent method for hospitals to adopt.

What services are required from biomedical technicians and clinical engineers? The biomedical technician, the clinical engineer, and the biomedical arm of the maintenance department must be concerned with safety of all electrical service devices, including those in patient and laboratory areas. They must also be concerned with equipment repair and service. This includes the calibration and repair of medical and laboratory equipment on a 7-day-a-week, 24-hour-a-day basis. Additionally, they must assist in providing specifications for procuring the equipment and become involved in setting up adequate preventive maintenance programs and maintenance record cards. The engineering department advises the hospital administration on JCAH, OSHA, state, and other regulatory agency involvement in the biomedical areas. And they should provide inservice education to the nursing and technical staffs in the hospital.

NOTES

1. U.S. Public Health Service, 1966, *The Hospital Laundry*, p. 7.

2. Ibid., p. 1.

3. Michael J. Shaffer, Joseph J. Carr, and Marian Gordon. "Clinical Engineering—An Enigma Health Care Facilities," *Hospital & Health Service Administration*, Summer, 1979, p. 77.

4. Ibid., p. 78.

5. Ibid., p. 80.

Chapter 14

Administrative Support Services

Key Terms

Purchasing agent ~ Prudent buyer ~ ABC analysis ~ Economic order quantity (EOQ) ~ Decentralized purchasing ~ Centralized purchasing ~ Full-time equiv-alents (FTEs) ~ Position control ~ Job description ~ Orientation program ~ Turnover rate ~ Taft-Hartley Act ~ Public Law 93-360 ~ Equal Employment Opportunity Act ~ Civil Rights Act ~ Age Discrimination in Employment Act ~ Auxiliary

PURCHASING DEPARTMENT

The hospital purchasing department is usually under the direction of a purchasing agent, a materials manager, or an assistant director of the hospital. Purchasing agent is a misnomer in some instances, since many of the goods purchased by the hospital may not be purchased through the purchasing department. For example, the pharmacy is for the most part responsible for the purchasing of drugs, and frequently the dietary department has a major hand in purchasing food for the hospital. This makes for a decentralized purchasing organization. However, generally, the purchasing agent has to determine what, when, and how much to purchase for hospital inventories. It is the purchasing agent who seeks out sources of supplies and proper vendors. The receipt of these goods and the receiving functions fall to the purchasing agent and personnel in the purchasing department. The purchasing agent is involved in authorizing receipts and invoices and comparing them with the specifications used upon ordering. The purchasing agent maintains a storeroom and issues merchandise from that storeroom. The purchasing department works very closely with the accounting department to maintain proper accounts payable records and inventory control. Occasionally, advanced purchasing departments will become involved in certain production research and in seeking out new products and testing them in the hospital. Hospitals, in varying degrees, have the opportunity to standardize their equipment and purchases. The purchasing agent is the key person in this process. On the other side of the equation, the disposal of furniture and equipment also usually passes through the purchasing agent. Finally, the purchasing agent must develop any written policies and procedures concerning the purchasing program.

The Purchasing Process and Competitive Bids

From the standpoint of the purchasing agent, the purchasing process begins when the vendors or salespersons acquaint the agent with their products. Generally, it is best to have the purchasing agent receive all salespersons and suppliers rather than have them approach the various departments.

The prudent buyer must be aware of the differences in pricing for various products purchased by the hospital. As cost containment becomes more important to federal agencies and third party payers, competitive bidding becomes vital. To obtain suitable bids, specifications for each product must be set down, preferably in writing. One of the side benefits for the hospital from competitive bidding is that the purchasing agent and the department heads who frequently request an item have to give more thought to the item, its usage, and the standards they require for it. One of the problems with using only price as a determinant is in the question of service. If the product needs repair, whether it be a major piece of equipment or a smaller disposable item, the purchasing agent must demand that the sales and service representatives for that vendor make good with a repair call or come in to discuss the product and its characteristics with the department heads. Service is an element that must be weighed along with price in competitive bidding. Notwithstanding the separate elements of service and quality, however, competitive bids are definitely successful economic tools for the purchasing agent and the hospital.

Inventories

Reviewers of hospital material management systems indicate that hospitals have lagged behind other manufacturing and retail industries in material management. This should be of some concern to the hospital administrator, since the cost of purchasing inventories and the management of those inventories represent a large and growing portion of the hospital's operating costs.

The hospital is a labor intensive industry with salaries and fringe benefits accounting for nearly 60 percent of all hospital operating expenses. During a recent ten-year period, when hospital payroll costs rose 236 percent, nonpayroll costs, including the cost of inventories and goods, rose 349 percent.[1] The major beneficiaries of these large increases in nonpayroll costs have been hospital vendors. Hospital suppliers have advanced arguments to explain why these increases have been so great. They indicate that the more sophisticated technology and clinical advances in the hospital have created an increased demand for a multiplicity of new products that were not in existence five years ago. The suppliers also point to the ever increasing use of disposables.

Hospitals must assess the capital that they use in relation to the purchasing process. One researcher estimates that the average hospital today carries an official inventory of approximately $630 per bed. Add to this amount the hospital's unofficial stocks that are charged off to operating expenses, and the total inventory of stocks approaches $1,000 per bed. Some experts believe that inventories of a magnitude of $1,000 per bed could be reduced by up to 50 percent if hospitals were more efficient. The nation's hospitals could save millions of dollars with improved, sophisticated purchasing and inventory management.

The purchasing agent has two tools available in the management of inventory control:

ABC analysis. The ABC classification system classifies the entire inventory in a hospital into three categories, based on the yearly dollar usage of the items in inventory. The high-dollar usage class is called A, the low dollar usage class is called C, and B items have a usage value that is somewhere between A and C.

In fact, the hospital spends most of its money on very few items. In a business retail firm, 80 percent of the business comes from 20 percent of the customers. Thus, in terms of hospital inventories, 80 percent of the cost might be spent on only 20 percent of the items in inventory.

Economic Order Quantity or EOQ Analysis. EOQ analysis determines the optimal audit quantities for a particular item in the hospital's storeroom. Using ABC analysis, the purchasing agent can then begin the task of determining the economical quantity of a particular item by class. First, the EOQ formula is used to calculate the annual usage of each item in dollars and then to determine the cost in dollars of placing the purchase order, the hospital's holding or carrying cost for the inventory, and the average inventory on hand at any given time. With this information, the purchasing agent can then make economic goals and efficient par levels for each inventory item. The hospital purchasing agent must reach a balance between the benefits realized from higher inventories and the cost of those inventories. Hospitals must come to grips with the cost and investment in inventory.

The Storeroom

The majority of the hospital's inventory is kept in the purchasing agent's hospital storeroom. Par levels or inventory records must be accurately maintained in the storeroom. There are literally hundreds of individual items in a given storeroom. The primary user of storeroom items is the nursing service department. The nursing units submit written lists of needed items to the storeroom, and the storeroom clerks package and place the stores on proper distribution carts. They are then delivered to the various nursing units and departments. Each of the items sent out of the storeroom as inventory is then charged to the proper internal accounting record, for example, the nursing unit. This is handled through interdepartmental accounting systems and the accounting office.

Purchasing Systems

Due to the nature of the dietary and pharmacy departments, hospitals have decentralized purchasing arrangements. There might be a centralized control of a centralized purchasing system, but in reality more and more of the items in the pharmacy are ordered by the pharmacist, and the same is true in the dietary area. If the hospital uses a decentralized purchasing system, it should at least center it on the large purchasing department rather than allow each department head from time to time to place orders with separate vendors.

There tends to be a belief that the more centralized the control and the more centralized the purchasing in a hospital, the more efficient the operation and the more cost containment can be realized by the hospital. A recent government report noted that "centralized purchasing is widely recognized as essential to cost containment programs. It can result in savings by consolidating the departmental needs and by reducing the number of employees involved in purchasing functions. Further, central purchasing provides the means for strengthening purchasing and for establishing clear purchasing policy."[2] The same government report stated that the greater the centralized management of purchasing in a hospital, the more the hospital can maximize its competition and the more easily it can participate in purchasing groups.[3]

Shared Purchasing

The concept of sharing purchasing power or group purchasing is not new to hospitals. Over the years, there have been experiments and cooperative arrangements. The purpose of these co-op arrangements is simply to reduce the cost of purchases to hospitals. Group purchasing can be as simple as two hospitals deciding to combine certain purchasing activities in order to obtain lower prices for goods or services. But one careful observer notes that there are "a host of different issues potentially arising out of shared purchasing arrangements. Any segment of shared services management that is colorably anticompetitive needs to be evaluated by antitrust standards in order to avoid costly and perhaps devastating litigation."[4] The reviewer suggested a competent legal counsel to examine any group purchasing arrangements.[5]

Leasing

Generally, in the purchase of capital equipment (and especially with the high cost of the highly technical and esoteric clinical equipment), administrators have been leasing equipment rather than purchasing it outright. In the last decade, the leasing of equipment by hospitals has grown enormously. The primary reason for this is that a lease offers the hospital (under Medicare reimbursement principles) faster reimbursement, since the lease can be a properly established expense. In addition, leasing allows administrators to purchase equipment without having the capital already in hand.

There are two types of leases: the financial lease and the operating lease. According to one expert on the subject, "the financial lease is a noncancellable contract. . . . Usually the term is no longer than 80% of the useful life of the asset."[6] The other type of lease is the operating arrangement, "in which the lessee may cancel the contract with due notice. Most copying equipment and highly technical medical equipment that may be subject to high degree of obsolesence are acquired through this type of lease. Again, reimbursement is based on retropayments."[7] Of course, under leasing arrangements, considering the time value of money, the hospital must bear the interest costs that are included in the lease payments.

Purchasing Practices

Hospitals purchase items in ways that, in some instances, are similar to the ways individual consumers purchase items; but, in other instances, the method is quite different. Individual consumers and hospitals both go through a rational process of identifying unsatisfied needs or wants, developing alternative ways of meeting these wants and needs, evaluating the alternatives, and finally reaching a purchasing decision. After purchasing the item, postpurchase behavior follows—either satisfaction or anxiety. Other similarities are: (1) Both find it at times difficult to effectively judge the quality of products. (2) Sometimes selection is restricted. (3) Very often, when a certain product or service is needed, we are not in a position to shop around for it. (4) There is sometimes an absence of price competition among the providers. (5) Much as we would like to believe it, hospitals and individuals are neither "rational buyers" nor classic "economic beings."

On the other hand, hospitals purchase in ways different from individuals. For example, the average hospital purchase is usually for a relatively few buying units compared to the consumer market. For example, there are only a little more than 7,000 hospitals, in contrast to 220 million consumers in 70 million households. There are other significant differences between hospital and individual purchasing: (1) The periods of negotiation in hospital purchasing are usually much longer. (2) The hospital market buys certain products very infrequently compared to the retail individual consumer. (3) The average hospital order may be considerably larger. (4) Direct sales from the producer to the individual consumer are rare, whereas in the hospital industry direct marketing from the producer to the industrial user or the hospital is more common. (5) In the hospital market, purchasing decisions are frequently influenced by more than one person; for example, the director of nursing who wants an item may discuss it with the assistant administrator, and together they may discuss it with the purchasing agent. (6) Catalog buying is much more prevalent among hospital users. (7) The hospital wants to purchase items based on excellent service records, considering the nature of the hospital business. (8) The hospital may insist upon adequate or more than adequate quality and on uniformity and standardization of products; this may not be as important in individual consumer purchases. (9) Hospitals can benefit through centralizing buying, since they buy so much and have greater purchasing power. (10) Group purchasing arrangements are much more common among hospitals than among individuals; the counterpart to a hospital purchasing group might be an individual joining a cooperative to buy groceries.

PERSONNEL DEPARTMENT

The hospital is a highly complex sophisticated industry, and it is the hospital staff that brings the institution to life. In the final analysis, the hospital is a place where people serve people. The selection and hiring of the personnel to work in the departments of the hospital are the responsibility of the management, the department heads, and the supervisors. However, it is the personnel department that coordinates these activities and assists the departments in their recruiting and selection needs.

There are several reasons for an organized personnel function: (1) Management has discovered that a well-functioning personnel department can bring economies of scale to the hospital operation. (2) It is psychologically important for the employees that one department oversee the maintenance and selection of personnel. (3) The personnel department is a strong administrative assistant to the management of the hospital, particularly now in view of the deluge of recordkeeping responsibilities placed upon personnel directors by the federal government and other regulatory agencies.

Department Functions

The basic functions in the personnel area include the employment process, an advisory capacity in the training and orientation of personnel, the important recordkeeping functions for the entire personnel area, and finally the coordination through a department of many of the people activities related to administration.

Unlike many of the hospital's departments, the personnel department is considered a staff support activity, as opposed to the line functions in the medical staff and in the departments of nursing, dietary, housekeeping, laundry, and maintenance.

The personnel department's activities are generally divided into two functional areas: obtaining employees, and maintaining those employees' records and programs once they are within the hospital organization.

Employment Functions

The first step in meeting the employment function is to understand and use an adequate position control plan. The position control plan is a tool of management that allows the hospital to control the number of full-time equivalent employees (FTEs) on the payroll compared to what was budgeted by administration. It generally falls to the personnel department to maintain the master files for position controls. The position control files include the title of the position, the number of positions, the salary scale for the division, and the authorized number of positions to be filled at any time. Each department head has a personnel section relating to the activity in that department and should maintain it as the personnel department does for the entire hospital.

Given the severe pressure from third party payers and federal government cost containment efforts, it is a major challenge to hospital management and the personnel department to provide high quality care while containing costs under a controlled staffing program or position control program. Effective position control programs based on approved personnel budgets and accurate records of employment will ensure hospital management control over the largest portion of the hospital's expense salaries and wages.

Before an employee can be recruited, selected, and brought into the hospital, the personnel department, in coordination with the department in which the employee will work, should conduct a job analysis. That is to say, the personnel department should observe and study the tasks and functions to be performed by the employee, the conditions under which the employee is supposed to work, the skills and training aptitude of the employee, and the requisite abilities necessary to perform the job.

Following the job analysis, a job description is drawn up. Job descriptions or specifications for jobs vary among hospitals. Generally, they include the job title, the work department, an outline of the tasks and duties to be performed, any equipment or special tools to be used, and the individual supervising the position. Each employee of the hospital should have a written job description. The description should be located in the personnel department, and the department head should be familiar with each one. The job description may include some job-related activities, such as educational experience, necessary special training, and certification required. It may even mention the salary code or salary range. One of the most extensive checks on job descriptions is in the publication *Job Descriptions and Organizational Analysis for Hospitals and Related Health Services, 1971,* published by the U.S. Department of Labor in cooperation with the American Hospital Association.

Another objective of the personnel department is to recruit good employees. Recruiting does not automatically happen; it requires work. There are several ways that a personnel department can obtain employees. The applicant might be a "walk-in" who simply comes into the personnel department and seeks employment. Another way—and an excellent method used by the author to fill vacant positions—is to recruit from within the hospital's employee ranks. It is a great morale booster to promote someone; there is no substitution for hiring a person already known to you.

Hospitals may also use the state employment offices, a source that is possibly more fruitful in large urban cities. For very special or difficult jobs, it may be necessary to use private employment agencies. Generally, the first level of screening is done by such an agency, and close adherence and conformity to a hospital's specifications for a certain task are an additional responsibility for the agency.

One of the easiest ways to seek applicants is through advertising in the mass media. Generally, hospitals have a great deal of experience with placing "help wanted" ads in local newspapers. However, this can be a very costly way to recruit if used too extensively. It also presents a real problem in screening applicants. The newspaper can be a "blind ad" where the job is mentioned but not the employer. An "open ad" allows the hospital employer to receive inquiries over the telephone and enables applicants to walk into the hospital.

After the personnel department has selected the best applicants, interviews are arranged and then the selection is made. It is strongly advised that, for a line position, the final choice of the applicant rest with the department head, the supervisor, or the assistant administrator. The personnel director should not make the final selection in most instances and should act only in an advisory capacity.

Once the employee is hired, the problems of retaining, motivating, and making the employee feel a part of the hospital begin. The orientation program can be helpful in retention. A simple method of employee orientation is to introduce the new employee to the hospital and his job.

An orientation has two basic purposes. First, it allows the new employee to gain background about the hospital and its functions and to see where the employee's job fits in. Second, the orientation should begin to make the employee feel a real part of the hospital. Any orientation program will have limitations and cannot be expected to solve magically all the problems that the employee will have. However, it certainly will aid in cutting down on confusion and lost time and in correcting money errors. For example, in the first month, 25 percent of the employee's time that would be spent on administrative matters can be saved. This can mean both a saving for the hospital and an increase in productivity.

Hospitals use different techniques in orienting employees. Some common techniques are a general orientation lecture, a general tour of the hospital, and distribution and explanation of the employee handbook. In some hospitals, the "buddy" system is used. Orientation time should be spent on the employee benefits program. The employee is particularly interested in questions of salary, the timing of salary payments, what additional benefits there are, and what the opportunities for promotion are.

Once the general orientation is over, it falls to the department head and to the supervisor to provide a more in-depth orientation about the department where the employee will be working. A very positive impression can be created if a follow-up to the orientation is conducted. Two or three weeks after the employee has been on the job, the personnel department could follow up by expressing an interest in the employee, seeing that the employee is adjusting well, and asking if there are any questions or problems. This makes common sense, is courteous, and can also improve the retention rate.

Training is different from formal education. In many hospital jobs, a certain required proficiency in the job specifications usually means that the employee should be already trained and proficient before starting the job. Basic training in hospitals includes: (1) informing the employee how to do the job as the hospital expects it, (2) demonstrating either in the classroom or in on-the-job training how to do it, (3) allowing the employee to do it (this could be called on-the-job training), and (4) critically advising the employee about mistakes and how performance might be improved. These aspects of training are common to many positions in the hospital—even if the employee already has a high level of proficiency in professional activities or a technical trade. For more formal, in-depth training, hospitals typically have well-organized training programs in the technical aspects of task-oriented nursing. For example, programs for nurse aides and nurse technicians have worked out very well in the hospital environment.

One of the measures that hospitals use to evaluate employee morale and retention is turnover. Personnel managers and department managers frequently are reminded if their turnover rate is too high. According to one observer, "turnover is generally defined to be that process in which employees leave employment at a given enterprise and cease to be counted as part of the payroll. But unless that employee is replaced he or she should not be counted as actual turnover."[8]

It is the personnel department's responsibility to maintain adequate records relating to turnover. As cost containment continues to be a major issue in hospitals, hospital managers will be looking carefully at the turnover rate. One reviewer has noted that "in the utilization of personnel one of the hidden costs is that of turnover. Various statistical studies have indicated an annual average turnover rate of more than 50 percent, as compared to about half that in all the U.S. business and industry. Costs are not easily determined, but estimates range from fifty dollars to one thousand five hundred dollars with an average of about three hundred dollars for each turnover.''[9] Clearly considering the high costs associated with turnovers, efforts should be made to maintain employees rather than allow them to leave employment.

The turnover rate is calculated by placing in the numerator the number of employees who were hired or left the payroll in a given month and by placing in the denominator the number of employees in the hospital. Turnover rates should be calculated every month. For example, if a hospital employed 25 new people in a given month, this would be placed over the total employee complement of, say, 400 employees, yielding a turnover rate for that month of 6.25 percent. Monthly turnover rates are summed for the 12 months of the year to obtain the annual turnover rate.

In the last two decades, hospitals have become very sensitive to the need to be competitive in their wage structures. It is generally understood that salary alone will not guarantee a loyal employee, quality productivity, or even retention in the hospital. However, with double digit inflation in our economy, salary is becoming more and more important, and the psychology of a salary is important for the personnel director to understand.

One knowledgeable expert put it this way: ''Men say that money talks. It does talk, but it has a strictly limited vocabulary. There are many things that salary cannot say; it cannot guarantee fair treatment. Even this statement that if a man has income enough he will do any job is not entirely true.''[10] Thus, even though wages are only one component of a compensation program, pressures have been mounting on hospitals over the last decade to increase their employees' wages and to improve their fringe benefit packages.

Hospitals generally consider certain factors when assigning a salary to an employee. These include the relative value and status of the job classification and job description. They also include a comparison of the current wage for similar work paid in nearby hospitals. In addition, the kind of work that is done on the job must be compared with competing industries in the same labor market.

Hospitals will pay employees based on their own institutional ability to generate cash and to meet the payroll. Another consideration is the need for exceptionally well-trained or exceptional persons. An illustration of this is the very high salaries paid to staff nurses by urban area hospitals that cannot attract nurses.

Increases in an employee's salary are usually based on periodic reviews and frequently involve employee appraisals and evaluations, usually by the department head or supervisor. Raises may be one of two kinds: (1) merit raises, by which employees are given increases based on their specific performances, and (2) standard or across-the-board raises that may be related somewhat to the cost of living. In the latter case, all employees receive the same percentage increase or a graduated percentage per-hour increase.

Fringe Benefits

Hospitals have traditionally offered benefits other than a paycheck in order to recruit and retain personnel. In years past, hospital wages were relatively low compared to those in industry, and it was common for hospitals to offer fringe benefits to compensate for low wages. Nowadays, with hospital salaries more competitive with industry, hospitals continue to offer fringe benefits. Some of the common fringe benefits that may be paid totally or partially by institutions include life insurance, group hospitalization, pension plans, and educational assistance. The payment of Social Security premiums is a standard fringe benefit. Also, some hospitals offer subsidized prices for meals and housing. Other institutions provide on-site recreational facilities for employees. The hospital should add the cost of providing these benefits to its salary and wage allotments in order to see the true picture of its labor costs.

Salary and Wage Administration

Over the last several years, there has been a great deal of pressure on hospitals, both from within the institution and from without, to control costs. Hospitals have had to review carefully the wages they pay. The personnel department has the job of developing, maintaining, and monitoring a salary wage program to aid in controlling costs.

The establishment of a salary and wage program includes four main steps:

1. Analyze each job, determining skills and education required for the job.
2. Place each job in a group or classification based on its relative importance to the hospital.
3. Assign a salary range to each classification.
4. Rate employees according to some system.[11]

Hospitals employ a variety of systems to rate employees. The rating scheme may involve a formal rating procedure based upon a supervisor filling out a form or completing a written report. The rating may be based on an employee's performance as ranked on a measured scale, or the rating could be based on the employee's performance as measured against an agreed-to set of standards. Regardless of the form taken, most hospitals find it necessary to construct some type of employee rating scheme.

Personnel Related to Nursing

As we have noted, the personnel department serves other departments of the hospital in an advisory capacity. It generally does not have what is known as line or operating authority. Yet, although the personnel director's relationship to department heads is advisory, the director must have direct access to top administration, even though the personnel recordkeeping functions and other roles may be under an assistant administrator. Since the personnel director's interpretation of personnel policies and statements can have an impact on the hospital, this officer must relate directly on many issues with the hospital administrator.

The centralized personnel administration function sometimes makes the relationship with the nursing department unclear. Nursing is the largest hospital department with a host of special job requirements. In dealing with the largest professional group of the hospital, the personnel department may find it difficult to handle directly the special or general problems concerning nursing. Some hospitals have set the professional nursing activities apart and have a subsidiary personnel office in the nursing department to recruit and maintain records on nurses. The hospitals that allow the personnel department to handle nursing problems and nursing personnel matters must have strong liaison arrangements, particularly in the recruiting, selection, and interviewing phases. Larger personnel departments may have nurse recruiters or nurse liaison individuals assigned to the personnel department. One of the strong connecting links between the nursing department and the personnel department is the exit interview of nursing personnel. The personnel department could retain a copy of the interview for future use in developing tactics for the recruitment and retention of nurses.

Hospitals and Unions

Unions within a hospital are an emotionally charged issue. Hospitals are a labor intensive industry that have, over the last decade, been challenged by unions and unionization moves. Those hospitals that are not unionized are constantly watching for any unionization activities. Yet the rumblings of the recent years are not the first indications of hospitals confronted by unions. The record shows that, as far back as 1919, there were instances of union activity in west coast hospitals. At that time, the *San Francisco Chronical* reported that five hospitals in that area attempted to organize to demand better working conditions and better working hours.[12] In 1936, the AFL-CIO initiated a unionizing campaign to organize hospitals. Their goal was to organize a significant portion of nonprofessional health care workers, including dietary, maintenance, and housekeeping personnel.

With the national growth in the union movement in the 1930s and the increased labor-related violence during that period, the federal government passed the Wagner Act in 1935. The Wagner Act stated the uniform rights of workers in their efforts to organize. In 1947, the Taft-Hartley Act or Labor-Management Relations Act was passed. This amended the Wagner Act with regard to the rights of management or employers; in addition, it also clarified the rights of labor. The employees of nonprofit hospitals were excluded from the provisions of the legislation. The reasons advanced for this exception vary, but generally it is believed that "the rationale focused on the fact that these institutions frequently assisted local government in carrying out their essential function and therefore should be left to exclusive local jurisdiction."[13] It is important to note that this interpretation was made in 1947, some 19 years before the enactment of Medicare and Medicaid programs, through which the government became deeply involved in the financing of health care. The exception of hospital employees under the Taft-Hartley Act did not mean that employees could not organize; it simply meant that, if they did organize, they did so without the protection of the federal government and the variety of laws that protected labor at that time.

Congress passed Public Law, 93-360 on July 26, 1974. This law removed the nonprofit hospital's exception from the Taft-Hartley Act. This meant that approximately 101 million unorganized employees in not-for-profit hospitals could be organized under the umbrella of the Taft-Hartley Act. Following the Taft-Hartley Act Amendments of 1974, the National Labor Relations Board (NLRB) categorized four labor units within hospitals: (1) registered nurses; (2) all other professionals, including interns, residents, and physicians on the medical staff; (3) service and maintenance employees, including business office employees; and (4) technical employees, including licensed practical nurses. The three largest health care unions at the present time are the American Federation of State, County, and Municipal Employees (AFSCME), the Services Employees International Union (SEIU), and the National Union of Hospitals and Health Care Employees.

Not surprisingly, hospital management has, for the most part, been opposed to the concept of labor organization within the hospital. One knowledgeable writer on the subject accurately represented hospital management's feelings by pointing out:

> The major consequence of a union is typically to lessen management's control in the utilization of personnel. The inability to make work assignments without jurisdictional disputes serves to swell the total pay and unions tend to swell the total payroll bill. In addition, promotions on seniority rather than merit basis can result in inefficient utilization of personnel. The possibility of difficulty in discharging ineffective personnel employees adds to the burden.[14]

With regard to the current unionization of hospital employees, a review shows that the percentage that is organized is somewhat less than that representing the total nonorganized work force. Of the total hospital employees, 14 percent are organized in all types of hospitals. The figure for employees of not-for-profit hospitals is somewhat less, 12.4 percent.[15]

To provide a defense against unions, the first thing a hospital ought to do is to review the principles it employs with regard to its employee programs and employee relations. The American Hospital Association has issued a statement on

"Employee Relations for Health Care Institutions." The Association indicates that the hospital should include in its policies and actions the following principles in dealing with employees:

- Policies should provide job security and job satisfaction.

- Employees should be offered opportunities for self-expression. The growth of the individual in skills, knowledge, mobility, and promotion should be defined in the hospital.

- Affirmative action programs and practices should be put into effect (in other words, nondiscriminatory selection and placement).

- Employees should be recognized for their accomplishments.

- All employees at all levels in the organization should be sensitive to making these principles work.

- Salaries, wages, and fringe benefits should be commensurate with standards in the marketplace.[16]

The professional registered nurse and physician have not been immune from union activity in hospitals. It is surely painful for older established nurses, physicians, and administrators to accept union organization of professional personnel. However, the old relationships that existed between nurses and physicians—more or less as partners in the management of the hospital and the care of the patient—seem to have gone. Following the 1974 Taft-Hartley Amendment, turbulences have broken out, and more and more registered nurses and physicians are talking about unionization or are actually unionizing. The record shows that to date only a relatively few nurses and physicians are unionized, but with the increased tensions in employee relationships and the drives by unions to bring in members, this percentage can be expected to increase.

Government Involvement

A hospital is unlikely to have had action taken against it because of its failure to comply with federal regulations on employment. However, personnel offices, administrators, employees, and members of the community should realize that there is, in fact, significant federal legislation that governs the selection, interviewing, and hiring processes in hospitals. The Civil Rights Act and the Equal Employment Opportunity Act of 1972 are geared to ensure that all employers, hospitals included, will not discriminate in their hiring opportunities and training based on race, color, religion, sex, or national origin. According to the civil rights legislation of 1964 (Title VII), this applies to all employer relationships concerning hiring, firing, wages, terms, and conditions or privileges of employment.

The Equal Employment Opportunity Commission (EOC) is the administrative and enforcement agency of Title VII. The EOC has stipulated general recordkeeping requirements for hospitals, as for other employers. For example, personnel or employment records must be kept by the employer. They must be preserved for at least six months, and the date the record was made or the personnel actions taken must be recorded. This also applies to many of the common records and forms in the department, such as application forms, layoff notices, and the like. To be in compliance with the Civil Rights Law, hospitals must be sincerely alert to discriminatory practices. Personnel directors, administrators, and hospital managers must review the interviewing process carefully to see that there is no discrimination in that area. They must also notify every employment agency they deal with that they are an equal opportunity employer. They must scrutinize carefully their wage structures to see that whites and minority group employees doing the same work are treated the same in compensation. In addition, the law forbids discrimination on the basis of sex. In short, hospitals should check out very carefully their employee facilities and privileges to be sure that there is no discrimination in the facilities, washrooms, cafeterias, and the like, based on civil rights conditions.

In 1963, the Equal Pay Act amended the Fair Labor Standards Act, known popularly as the Federal Wage and Hour Law. This is another federal legislative act that personnel directors must be acutely aware of. It was designed primarily to protect women from being discriminated against with respect to wages. Specifically, it prohibits hospitals from paying different or lower wages to a woman who is performing the same job as a male counterpart. Many states have also enacted equal pay laws. In compliance with the Wage and Hour Law, the hospital must provide the wage-and-hour administration with adequate records concerning the different occupations and job specialties in the hospital, specifying which categories are filled by male and female persons. These records normally have to be retained for two years.

In 1967, Congress passed the Age Discrimination in Employment Act. This is federal legislation that prohibits employers or companies with more than 25 people from discriminating against personnel who happen to be more than 40 years old and less than 65 years old. Again, the federal government requires records to be kept and certain posters to be displayed throughout the hospital. The enforcement of the age discrimination law parallels very closely the enforcement requirements of the federal wage-hour law. Once again, more than 50 percent of the states have also banned discrimination based on age. However, as one might imagine, these laws are not as uniform as the federal law.

If the Equal Employment Opportunity Commission were to find a hospital or any employer in violation of the federal Civil Rights Act, it is likely that the hospital would be asked to produce an affirmative action plan. According to one source, "an affirmative action plan has been defined as an organization's positive remedy for problems that create inequality or lack of equal opportunity within its total employment structure."[17] It is important to realize that, at least for now, the Office of Federal Contract Compliance (OFCC), the agency of the government that administers the affirmative action plan, has not required hospitals to produce such plans simply on the basis of participating in the federal Medicare program.

All of these laws impact upon selection procedures in the personnel department. The essence of the selection procedure is to provide the hospital with the highest quality, best trained, and most adaptable employees. Given the battery of federal legislative acts, rules, and executive orders, personnel directors must be sensitive to indicators, such as age, sex, marital status, and others that have been used in the past. It is possible that a review of the personal characteristics of applicants done years ago might be in violation of Title VII of the Civil Rights Act.

Occupational Licensure

With the ever-increasing application of new medical and scientific discoveries, additional pressures have been mounting on health manpower resources. Sophisticated diagnostic and treatment methods require that the established health professions expand their roles. Governments have recognized the emergence of the new health care professionals by (1) acknowledging their creation and (2) trying to superimpose on the professions some sort of occupational licensure system that requires the emerging professionals or technicians to demonstrate a competence in the field before they receive a license to practice.

For example, the state of Pennsylvania has reviewed the matter of licensure for the new health professionals and concluded:

> The legislative acts defining the scopes of practice have created a troublesome fragmentation and an increasingly integrated set of services, while specifying rigid restrictions on the methods which may be employed in the delivery of health care. Two major criticisms of the existing occupational license system in the recent years extend directly from the fragmentation and those rigidities: (1) Emergency and proliferation of regulated specialities have created a system so complex and so cumbersome that the flexibility to the most efficiently and economically operated health care introduces additional cost to the consumer and (2) The current system restricts vertical and lateral occupational mobility for the health care professional.[18]

Clearly, one of the major criticisms against rigid licensure, particularly with respect to the newer professions, is that increased regulation will only serve to choke off innovations in the health care area. Though many astute observers believe that the fragmented licensing system in the health care community that exists today is wanting, there seems to be no general consensus on how to replace or restructure it.

A selected list of health occupations within the hospital is provided in Appendix A. The list includes a brief description of the profession or technical role, with a code following the description indicating the level of education required for the position. It also includes addresses to write to for further information on particular disciplines.

VOLUNTEERS

Hospital volunteers fall into two general groups. One group, usually referred to as hospital volunteers, works primarily in the functional areas of the hospital; the second group works primarily outside the hospital in activities not related to the functions of the hospital. People in this group are referred to as auxiliaries or women's auxiliaries, grey ladies, candy stripers, or guilds. The hospital volunteer provides free services to the hospital. A review of the records shows that there are 37 million volunteers in the United States. Of these, 59 percent are women and 41 percent are men. It is estimated that volunteers give 3.5 million hours of service per year, an estimated dollar volume of 33.9 billion dollars. It is interesting that this sum is almost equal to the annual budget of the Department of Health, Education and Welfare.[19]

The Role of Volunteers

There was a time when the hospital volunteer was restricted to the women's auxiliary in work at the hospital snack bar or in visits to patients with a hospitality cart. Those days have passed. The women's auxiliary continues to staff gift shops and snack bars, and this hospitality is still needed. However volunteers have now entered all aspects of the functioning of the hospital. Their mission is to supplement the services provided by the hospital's employees. Volunteers are found operating switchboards, aiding families and friends at the reception desk, and serving as volunteer patient representatives. They may provide nursery service on a day-care basis. They aid the social service department by listening to the terminally ill; they perform puppet shows for the children in the pediatric unit. They may be transportation aides in the x-ray or physical therapy departments. Many of them aid the management of the hospital by offering skilled typing services and clerical skills.

The auxiliary services based outside the operating functions of the hospital get involved in gift shop work or snack bar operations, but they also become more directly involved in fund-raising activities. They constitute a strong community-relations arm of the hospital.

The Typical Volunteer

Barbeito and Hoel have identified and characterized the traditional hospital volunteer in the following way:

> The traditional volunteer has been the white, middle-class, married woman between the ages of 25 to 44 whose available time is often limited by family demands. She has frequently rendered her services to obtain social status and recognition for herself or to assist her husband or children. Her male counterpart is the volunteer who works in upper or mid-level management or in other professional positions whose voluntary activity often serves to enhance his employment situation.[20]

This is a traditional view of volunteers, and the truth is that it is breaking down, in part due to the influence of the feminist movement in this country. The National Organization for Women has spoken out strongly against the exploitation of women through volunteerism.

Volunteer Department

There is no single way to organize the volunteer department. The JCAH is skimpy in its reference to volunteers in the hospital. According to its Standard V, "if volunteer services are to be used, volunteers shall be trained and supervised. Volunteers who provide professional services shall meet the same requirements of qualifications and performances as applied to paid staff. Supportive personnel and technical assistants shall be appropriately supervised and their duties shall be specified."[21]

The key aspect of the organization of volunteers is the volunteers' authority in the hospital. Generally this authority is recognized in the hospital's bylaws. The bylaws delineate the functions and purposes of the volunteer effort. The volunteer department in the hospital is usually headed by a director of volunteers who may be a salaried full-time individual. This individual generally reports to the assistant administrator or perhaps to the administrator of the hospital. Frequently, the hospital's auxiliary is a guild affair with its own auxiliary officers. In some instances, the auxiliary is a volunteer department, but it is more common to have a separate auxiliary and inhospital volunteer service.

Director of Volunteers

If the hospital has a volunteer service, there is a director of volunteers, either part-time or full-time, depending on the extent of the volunteer program. This individual is responsible for recruiting volunteers, interviewing them, arranging their assignments with various functional department heads in the hospital, providing their orientation, and assisting in training. The director is also responsible for maintaining a strong liaison with the functional department heads with whom the volunteers work and relate. It is the director's job to keep the volunteers informed of pertinent hospital policies and procedures. The volunteer director should recruit based on a reasonable level of hospital need, balancing the recruitment of teenagers and more mature adults against the needs of the hospital. Sometimes in the recruitment of volunteers the hospital's own employee staff and members of the board of directors and their families are overlooked as potential volunteers. In some cases, the auxiliary of the hospital can provide resources for the inservice volunteer department as well as the auxiliary by drawing from the members of the inservice volunteer department as recruits. In choosing volunteers, consideration must be given to the potential volunteer's motivation for service. The director must match the volunteers' characteristics of maturity, stability, and dependability in the function to which they are assigned.

Volunteers' Orientation

Once volunteers have been selected, it falls to the director of volunteers and the hospital management to place them into a productive position. Volunteers should not feel lost in the environment. They should have the opportunity to understand the mission of the hospital, be acquainted with the functions of the hospital and how it operates, just as any employee would. Volunteers should be assigned tasks in the department in which they are able to perform. Generally, volunteers provide many extra services in addition to the regular and essential tasks provided by the hospital's paid employees. These include reading and writing for patients, delivering mail, assisting in making beds, and escorting patients and visitors.

The orientation program sponsored by the director of volunteers can feed upon the employee orientation program. Sometimes the volunteers can make valuable suggestions for improvements in the hospital, since they frequently bring new perspectives from their prior experience. Once volunteers have selected a job and been assigned, they expect some minimal amount of on-the-job training. It is reasonable to expect the employees in the department with whom the volunteer is working to show an interest in the volunteer, just as any fellow employee would be treated. Volunteers should expect to be supervised and treated like all other workers within the department.

Ethical and Legal Implications

Hospital volunteers should seek to serve charitable institutions or needy patients. However, even in for-profit hospitals, caution should be used to make it clear that the volunteer effort is not being used to improve the profits of the institution. In addition, there are certain ethical implications concerning volunteers who might replace paid employees of the hospital. This can become particularly agitating in an area of high unemployment. According to the U.S. Fair Labor Standards Act (Wage and Hour Law), the placing of a volunteer in a position as a typist or in an open employee position establishes a legal employee-employer relationship that violates the spirit of the law and the spirit of volunteerism. The American Hospital Association seeks to have volunteers perform supplementary tasks that will contribute to the well-being and comfort of hospitalized patients, tasks that are of great importance but that are not normally performed by regular hospital employees, so that employees' jobs will not be in jeopardy.

Though hospitals do not strive to place volunteers in the legal position of hospital employees, hospitals must realize that, when volunteers are acting on behalf of the hospital, according to the law they are in a master-servant relationship with the institution. Accordingly, the hospital is responsible for the volunteer's acts that are performed in the line of duty. Not only is the hospital responsible for the volunteer's actions, it is also responsible for preventing the volunteer from becoming involved in tasks or jobs beyond the volunteer's capacity. A wise hospital manager will ensure protection for the hospital by maintaining a proper insurance policy that covers the volunteers in case of accidental injury on the job or injury to a patient, staff member, or visitor.

Benefits for the Hospital

Aside from the fact that hospitalized patients may enjoy a friendly cheerful face and a visit from a volunteer, the hospital reaps other benefits from volunteer effort. Volunteers provide an excellent way to communicate between the hospital and the community. Volunteers can be indispensable in a fund-raising campaign. In times of difficulty within the hospital, whether it be labor problems or other unforeseen circumstances, volunteers are frequently used to augment the nonskilled labor force.

Volunteers are a special source of strength and support to the hospital. Throughout this country's brief history, they have offered service to millions of hospital patients. Let us hope that volunteerism in the country as a whole and particularly within the health care arena does not wane and that hospital management is able to structure new and challenging roles for the hospital volunteer.

NOTES

1. I. Donald Snook, Jr., "Controlling Inventory on the Emergency Room," *Hospital Financial Management*, March 1979, p. 34.

2. U.S. General Accounting Office, 1979, *Study of Purchasing and Materials Managenent Functions in Private Hospitals*, Part I, p. 4.

3. Ibid., pp. 4-5.

4. Andrew K. Dolan, "What Are the Antitrust Implications of Shared Purchasing for Hospitals? " *Hospitals, JAHA*, October 16, 1979, p. 76.

5. Ibid.

6. James B. Henry, "Know Your Lease," *Hospitals, JAHA*, August 16, 1974, p. 64.

7. Ibid.

8. Frank Murphy, *Personnel Administration Handbook for Hospitals and Health Institutions* (Fond du Lac, Wisc.: HPA and Co., 1961), p. 22.

9. Malcolm T. MacEachern, *Hospital Organization and Management* (Chicago, Ill.: Physicians Record Co., 1957), p. 265.

10. Norman D. Bailey, *Hospital Personnel Administration* (Berwyn, Ill.: Physicians Record Co., 1959), p. 187.

11. Murphy, *Personnel Administration Handbook*, p. 82.

12. *San Francisco Chronicle*, 1919.

13. Norman Metzger and Dennie D. Pointer, *Labor Management Relations in the Health Care Industry: Theory and Practice* (Washington, D.C.: Science and Health Publications, Inc., 1969), p. 49.

14. Jonathan S. Rakich, Beaufort B. Longest, Jr., and Thomas R. O'Donovan, *Managing Health Care Organizations* (Philadelphia, Pa.: W.B. Saunders Co., 1977), p. 14.

15. Rockwell Schulz and Alton C. Johnson, *Management of Hospitals* (New York, N.Y.: McGraw-Hill Book Co., 1976), p. 245.

16. American Hospital Association, "Employee Relations for Health Care Institutions" (Chicago, Ill.: AHA, 1975).

17. Rakich, Longest, and O'Donovan, *Managing Health Care Organizations*, p. 214.

18. Hospital Educational and Research Foundation of Pennsylvania, *Alternate Regulations of Health Personnel* (Camp Hill, Pa.: AHA, 1976), p. 1.

19. Brandy Rommel, "Confrontation with Change: 1976 Review of Literature," *Volunteer Leader* 18, no. 2 (Spring 1978): 29-35.

20. Carol L. Barbeito and Robert Hoel, "Recruitment: A Supermarket of Volunteers," *Volunteer Leader* 19, no. 1 (Spring 1978): 30-36.

21. Joint Commission on Accreditation of Hospitals, *Accreditation Manual for Hospitals—1980 Edition* (Chicago, Ill.: JCAH, 1979), p. 50.

Chapter 15

Patient Support Services

Key Terms

Dietician ≈ Nutritionist ≈ Conventional system ≈ Convenience food ≈ Cool chill system ≈ Frozen ready ≈ Special diets defined ≈ Almoner ≈ Social worker ≈ Quality assurance ≈ Discharge planning

DIETARY DEPARTMENT

No department in the hospital reaches more patients, hospital staff, and visitors than the dietary department. If the food service is good and adequate, it receives only faint praise from patients and personnel. If the food service is inadequate, criticisms abound. Complaining patients often say, "For what I am paying for this room, you would think that the food would be better. It could be hot. I could have it when I want it, and if I want a cup of coffee, I should be able to get it at any time." These comments speak to the crucial public relations aspect of the dietary department.

The dietary department has a role in the therapeutic care of the patients as well as in providing standard food menus for the patients and staff. Every hospital should have a qualified professional dietician (concerned with planning and directing the food and meal service) and a nutritionist (involved in teaching patients about nutrition). This is the therapeutic aspect of a dietary department. Much of the department's efforts, however, are devoted to the preparation and feeding of patients and personnel. This tends to be a management and logistical function.

In earlier times, the preparation and delivery of food were under the auspices of either the nursing department, the head housekeeper, or the chief cook. Then the

157

housekeeping department underwent an evolution, and the dietary department started to take on a separate entity and was removed from the nursing service area. Developments in the world of nutrition and dietetics had an impact on the formation of special dietary departments. The medical profession began to look at the role of proper diet and nutrition as an aid to maintaining good health. A second development was in the evolution of the dietary profession itself. The dietary profession, through its membership in the American Dietetic Association, numbers over 14,000 people. The American Dietetic Association has given emphasis to the sophisticated training of dieticians and nutritionists. The Association prescribes a dietetic internship of three years of supervised work experience for its members.

There are two positions related to the dietary area that are common in hospitals. One is the dietician. Dieticians are primarily responsible for feeding the hospital patients and the staff. They are professionally educated individuals with advanced degrees. The second position is that of the nutritionist. The nutritionist is an individual educated in the science of nutrition and is primarily involved in educational and teaching programs within the hospital. The nutritionist plays an active role in patient therapy, both for inpatients and outpatients, and works closely with physicians and patient education programs. The nutritionist may also be involved in research.[1]

Patient Menus

It is the dietician's responsibility to plan menus for the patients and staff. The hospital dietician must have sound technical knowledge about foods as well as sufficient imagination to group foods attractively for meals. Dieticians must be sensitive to the psychological impact that food can have on the well-being of patients. In the past, hospitals were known as institutions serving questionable quality of food, but today's hospitals find themselves catering more to the patients' needs and wants, as well as to their nutritional needs. They offer a selection of meats, vegetables, and desserts, including out-of-season products and hothouse fruits.

Dieticians prefer two- or three-week schedules in preparing their menus. Basic outlines are used, and daily adjustments are made to handle special diet needs. The selective menu in hospitals has gained wide acceptance and use. As might be expected, the selective menu is easier to implement in the larger hospitals. Menus are modified by having the dietician regularly visit the patients to determine their needs and wants. The public relations aspect of a dietician's visit cannot be underestimated. Improving the nutritional services by reducing patient complaints and making the patients feel they are special is a crucial part of the hospital dietician's role.

Type of Food Service

Because of the increasing pressure on hospital management to contain costs, and because of the demands and wants of patients and the changing state of the art in food service, hospitals have recently been exploring a variety of different methods to produce and deliver high-quality meals. There are basically four types of services in the preparation and delivery of food in hospitals: the conventional system, the convenience food system, the cook-chill system, and the frozen ready (cook freeze) system. Food service experts describe the four systems as follows:

> The conventional system is the system which uses a menu prepared from basic ingredients daily with preparation assembly and finishing accomplished on the premises.
>
> The convenience system is the system which uses menu items that for the most part have been commercially prepared off the premises and then have been frozen and/or freeze dried in a form that can be easily prepared on site without the need for anything more complex than simple heating. An example of this type of item is the preplated hospital special diet meal similar to the TV dinner.
>
> The cook-chill system is the system which entails the use of on-site prepared products that are not necessarily utilized the day of preparation; they are flash-chilled, stored in the chill state (about 35 degrees F.), and reheated just prior to service.
>
> The frozen ready (cook-freeze) food system is a system which uses primarily a menu that is mass-produced on site, frozen, and stored in a form that requires only tempering (thawing), and reheating before service.[2]

The hospital could select a combination of these four systems for its particular production system. Studies have shown that exclusive use of one of the systems has defects that cause problems in the working of the system. Selection among the four systems is, of course, left to the dietician and to the hospital manager. The cost—the operating cost per meal and the annual cost per meal—varies from 40 to 50 cents per meal between the least expensive and the most expensive meal. The convenience system tends to be the highest cost, and the conventional system tends to be at a lower cost per meal.

Depending on the method of food production the hospital selects, the tracers to the patients will vary. But essentially there are two basic systems of tracers: the centralized and the decentralized. Many hospitals have modifications of each of these systems, due to the physical layout of the hospital. The bulk food delivery system is really a hybrid of the centralized and decentralized systems.

The centralized system is used by many hospitals because it provides for greater efficiency, economy, and supervision as well as efficient utilization of personnel time. Patient trays are centrally prepared and checked under central supervision along a conveyor belt, somewhat like an assembly line in an automobile industry. The decentralized system is the oldest method of serving food. In the decentralized system, the food is prepared and placed on the patients' trays in substations of the nursing units. This is a less efficient means than the centralized system. Because each nursing unit needs a separate kitchen for the distribution of food, capital costs are increased. One of the weaker links in the centralized food system may be the act of getting the tray to the patient's bedside. Since the trays are brought to the nursing unit in large carts, the food may lose heat or become less cold in transit.

Special Diets

There is an increasing use of special diets for hospital patients. This has occurred because of advances in diet therapy and a greater understanding of nutrition. Special diets are actually based on physicians' therapeutic orders that are placed in the patient's medical records. A physician, in consultation with the dietician or nutritionist, will recommend a specific diet based on a patient's condition. Special diets for patients are prepared under the direct supervision of a responsible dietician or nutritionist. Since the variety of food may be greatly reduced, it poses a real psychological challenge for the dietician to make the special tray attractive and eye-appealing.

Another member of the dietary team is the food service manager who works under the supervision of the administrative dietician. The manager supervises and instructs employees working in the food preparation area, the cafeteria, and coffee shop.

Physical Facilities

The physical facilities of the food preparation area involve more than just a kitchen. The dietary area must have a method of receiving the foodstuffs. Thus, a receiving area and platform and an administrative area are necessary. In addition, once the food is on the premises, it is important to see that there is clean and appropriate storage. There should be a central storage area, both dry storage and refrigerator storage. Further, the food production area must be close to the storage area to reduce the people cost and the cost of transporting the food to the area. In the food preparation area, there are cooking and baking facilities. Numerous broilers, friers, and ovens should be available. There is also a dishwashing area.

The employee cafeteria, which provides cafeteria service for the hospital staff, the medical staff, visitors, and even ambulatory hospital patients, is under the jurisdiction of the dietary department. Two elements in the cafeteria area are the serving lines and the dining area. There was a time when hospital cafeterias essentially offered subsidized food as a fringe benefit; this allowed hospitals to rationalize lower salaries. As hospital employees' salaries have become more competitive, hospital cafeteria prices have also risen.

The hospital cafeteria is usually near the food preparation area, so that service elevators or dumbwaiters can aid in transporting the food from the food preparation area to the cafeteria. Hospitals usually serve at least three meals a day; in some hospitals, a midnight meal is also served. Sometimes, hospitals supplement their hospital cafeteria with food and beverage vending machines. It is frequently the dietary department's responsibility to oversee the hospital's vending operations. The chronic problem in these areas is, of course, the housekeeping, which becomes the problem for the housekeeping department.

Contract Food Services

As hospitals continue to explore different methods of delivering and preparing food, they have also been exploring dietary department contract services. The American Hospital Association defines contract services as "a departmental management contract considered to be a formal agreement between a health care institution and a contractor under which the contractor is to provide the institution various management functions and which may include other services in return for a fee."[3]

An increasing number of hospitals engaged outside management for their dietary and food area, usually relying upon commercial retail sources for this purpose. The results range from quite satisfactory to unsatisfactory. However, on balance, contract food services can do a satisfactory job. There are pros and cons to hospital food management contract services. Some of the advantages of having an outside contracting service include the use of highly specialized trained personnel from an outside source, thereby reducing the need for hospital personnel. Indeed, the outside service may provide specialized personnel that the hospital does not have. Further, the outside management group may reduce costs through improved methods and efficiency. The byproduct of this may be a lower personnel staff in the dietary area, depending on the method of food service selected. This could free up space formerly occupied by food preparation equipment in the hospital and allow room for other departments. It also permits the hospital to review regularly the performance of the outside management.

Outside contractors would list, as their advantages, higher productivity, outstanding supervision, increased administrative interest, the provision of advanced equipment products, and research on food systems. They would make the point that outside contractors bring more flexibility to the hospital's changing scene. On the other side of the ledger, there are advantages for the hospital in maintaining their own inhouse services. One advantage is employee loyalty, that is, employees who are paid by the hospital may be more loyal. Moreover, hospitals have found that, with full-time employees of the hospital, a certain scheduling flexibility may be achieved. Also, a spirit of teamwork is generated by having the hospital use its own dietary department and by having its dietary employees work with other departments. Some hospitals would argue that, by having all the employees under their jurisdiction, security will be increased. Still, the proprietary food companies have a definite vested interest in offering their services at competitive prices and have proven themselves to be as efficient and effective as possible in order to retain the hospital's contract as long as possible.

Relationship with Nursing

Since the dietary department is also a therapeutic service and its activities relate for the most part to the patients on the nursing units, the maintenance of good working relationships with the nursing service department is absolutely critical if the dietary department is to complete its job successfully. Since both departments are concerned with therapy and their functions are interlocked, they must conduct their jobs in harmony or else confusion will reign and the patient will suffer. Sometimes the nursing staff must supplement the dietary department. This might occur if a special tray must be brought to the nursing unit for a patient who has just been admitted or if something special must be sought from the dietary department. Indeed, the nursing service department is the "eyes" of the nutritionist and dietician on the floor. If a patient is not eating well or other problems arise with the food, it is up to the nurse to keep the dietician informed. The dietician must read nursing notes and physicians' orders on the patient's chart to determine the proper diet.

SOCIAL SERVICE DEPARTMENT

Dr. Malcolm MacEachern, the established father of hospital administration, notes in his classic textbook, *Hospital Organization and Management,* the nineteenth century British hospital had the equivalent of our social worker, called an "almoner." According to MacEachern, the almoner was the individual who represented the community that dispensed alms. The almoner's chief duty was to prevent the abuse of charity. The almoner was also involved deeply in the social programs of the hospital. MacEachern traces this individual from the moralistic almoners of the Middle Ages, noting that the nineteenth century British counterpart had very little of the true spirit of charity. Apparently, the almoner's chief objective was the offering of aid but with the expenditure of as little money as possible. Whatever the merits of the nineteenth century almoner, this individual appears to have been the forerunner of the present-day social worker in the hospital.

America's first organized social service department in a hospital was formed by Dr. Richard C. Cabot at the Massachusetts General Hospital in 1905. At that time, the social worker was a brand new means of complementing the efforts of physicians in delivering better medical care. Dr. Cabot's projected role for the newly formed profession was "to investigate and report to the doctor domestic and social conditions bearing on diagnosis and treatment, to fill the gap between his orders and their fulfillment and to form the link between the hospital and the many societies, institutions and persons whose deed could be enlisted."[4]

Today, the JCAH notes the following in connection with hospital social service work: "Social work services shall be well-organized, properly directed, staffed with a sufficient number of qualified individuals, and appropriately integrated with other units and departments/services of the hospital."[5]

Qualifications of a Medical Social Worker

Social workers in the social service departments are highly trained individuals. Specifically, they must have graduated from a baccalaureate program, and may have taken advanced training at the master's degree level. The American Association of Medical Social Workers has set down the qualifications of training and eligibility for membership in that organization.

Functions of the Department

The modern day hospital can expect the social service department to make six specific contributions to the mission of the hospital:

1. to aid the health team to understand the social, economic, and emotional factors that affect the patient's illness, treatment, and recovery
2. to aid the patient and the patient's family to understand these factors and to make constructive use of the resources in the medical care system
3. to promote the well-being of the patient and improve the patient's family's morale by working with the family and the patient
4. to improve the mission of the hospital by becoming involved in hospital education and activities with the hospital staff and members of the outside community
5. to offer better patient care by making various services, including those outside the hospital, available to the patient
6. to improve the utilization of the community's resources and to impact these resources in order to aid patient and family needs when the patients leave the hospital.

One observer, in analyzing the extent to which the social worker can affect the patient and the patient's recovery, commented:

> The extent to which the patient is ready to accept advice from the social worker is dependent on two points: 1. the degree to which his physician sees the need for advice from the social worker and 2. the patient's understanding of the services of the social workers. They found that the physician's understanding not only of the social and emotional factors in relation to the care of a particular individual, but also his understanding of the functions and skills of the social worker and being of service to his patient, definitely reflects the degree to which the Social Service Department is dependent. The department is used by the physician in the care of his patient. The awareness of the physician of this service is the important criterion in determining the effectiveness of the social services.[6]

The important point is that if social service is truly to be effective, it must be directly related to communication with the physician and the patient.

A New Role for the Medical Social Worker

Since the American Hospital Association launched its Quality Assurance Program (QAP) and the federal government, through its PSROs, has been pushing for quality assurance programs for hospitals, the social worker has taken on an important role in aiding the process of quality assurance. The social worker has been an important functioning member of the hospital's utilization review committee. The JCAH has mandated that "the hospital shall demonstrate appropriate allocations of its resources through an effective utilization review program."[7]

As a committee member on the quality assurance program of a hospital, the social worker's most important contribution is in the area of discharge planning. The JCAH recommends that the social service department have a written policy and procedure for discharge planning. Discharge planning is the organized, centralized system to ensure that each hospitalized patient has a planned program to provide the needed continuing care and follow up the patient requires. Physicians, nurses, and administrators frequently look to the social worker to aid in arranging programs to enable patients to receive continuing care after they leave the hospital environment.

One of the social worker's crucial roles is to find an extended-care bed or a rehabilitation hospital bed for the patient who is unable to go home. In this task, the medical social worker impacts directly not only on the patient's well-being but also on the cost effectiveness and efficiency of the hospital's operations. If the patient is moved into a nursing home bed, the hospital runs a risk of losing reimbursement.

Thus, willingly or not, the social worker in the hospital environment has become an agent of the administration and the financial manager in saving the hospital money.

Beyond that, the medical social service department may yield benefits that are quite intangible. Though unmeasured in dollars, these benefits are reflected in the comments of the patients and their families that the social workers serve. Hospitals have found that medical social service departments have become an indispensible element in the hospital organization. Physicians frequently add their praise for the medical social worker, indicating their great contribution to the rapid rehabilitation of patients.

NOTES

1. Joseph K. Owen, *Modern Concepts of Hospital Administration* (Philadelphia, Pa.: W.B. Saunders Co., 1962), p. 409.
2. Matthew L. Herz and James J. Souder, Jr., "Preparation Systems Have Significant Effect on Costs," *Hospitals, JAHA,* January 1, 1979, p. 89.
3. American Hospital Association, "Departmental Management Contracts," *Technical Advisory Bulletin, Modern Concepts,* 1979, p. 1.
4. Owen, *Hospital Administration,* p. 320.
5. Joint Commission on Accreditation of Hospitals, *Accreditation Manual for Hospitals—1980 Edition* (Chicago, Ill.: JCAH, 1979), p. 177.
6. George P. Berry, ed., *Readings in Medical Care* (Chapel Hill, N.C.: University of North Carolina Press, 1958), p. 245.
7. Joint Commission on Accreditation of Hospitals, *Accreditation Manual,* p. 193.

Part VII

Hospital Finances

Chapter 16

Generating Revenue

Key Terms

Third party payer ~ *Public Law 89-97* ~ *Title XVIII and XIX* ~ *Medicare Part A and Part B* ~ *Reasonable Cost* ~ *Medically indigent* ~ *Fund accounting* ~ *General fund* ~ *Hill-Burton obligations* ~ *Profit and loss statement* ~ *Balance sheet*

INTRODUCTION

The principal difference between the economics of hospitals and that of retail businesses that we are all familiar with lies in how the hospital receives payment for its services to the patient. In the majority of cases, the hospital does not receive payment directly from the patient for the services rendered but rather from a third party payer. A third party is "any agent other than the patient who contracts to pay all or part of a patient's hospital bill."[1]

TYPES OF THIRD PARTY PAYMENTS

Patients can be classified by the following four methods of third party payment: Medicare, Medicaid, Blue Cross, and self pay or other insurance.

Medicare

On July 1, 1966, Public Law 89-97, the Medicare program became effective across the nation. The Medicare program was an outgrowth of a federal legislative process to meet the growing problems of the aged and the disabled in receiving appropriate health services that they could afford. As part of the Social Security

Amendments of 1965 (commonly referred to as Title XVIII), Medicare benefits were provided to senior citizens (over the age of 65) under two separate but closely related programs. These programs are referred to as Part A of Title XVIII, which pays for hospital services as well as nursing home care and other institutional care, and Part B of Title XVIII (known as Supplementary Medical Insurance), which basically pays for physician fees and certain diagnostic services. The supplementary program, or Part B, is voluntary. After age 65, the beneficiary can subscribe to this at a nominal cost.

Payment to the hospitals from Medicare is usually made directly. The basis for this payment is "reasonable cost." Reasonable cost is determined through a very elaborate cost-finding process called the cost report, which is prepared by the hospital at the end of its fiscal year. Costs not generally acceptable to third parties are any costs not directly related to the care of patients.[2]

Since its passage in 1966, Medicare has become generally very popular with consumers. For the average patient, there are four distinct pluses in the Medicare program:

1. It provides almost universal coverage for the elderly.
2. It offers far better benefits than any private health insurance program could offer to this age group.
3. It assures senior citizens a certain level of access to quality care institutions.
4. It requires relatively small out-of-pocket expenses for the elderly to be covered by the insurance.

So much for the pluses of Medicare. What about the minuses? They can be summed up in a single phrase: excessive costs. In the sober words of a Senate committee on the financing of Medicare studies: "The Medicare and Medicaid programs are in serious financial trouble. The two programs are also adversely affecting health care costs in financing for the general population."[3]

Medicaid

Along with Medicare legislation in 1966, Medicaid legislation was enacted under the Title XIX. The primary purpose of the Medicaid legislation was to finance health care services for the poor and medically indigent. However, unlike Medicare which was universally applied to all citizens over the age of 65, it was left to each of the 50 states to determine who were "needy" or medically indigent and thus eligible for Medicaid benefits. Each state designed its own health services benefit plan. Thus, the Medicaid program is administratively handled at the state level.

Typically, the costs of the Medicaid program are shared by the federal government and the individual states on an approximately 50-50 basis. Hospitals are reimbursed for inpatient services on the basis of "reasonable cost" as they are under Medicare; however, each of the states can define its own reasonable costs. The big discrepancy in the Medicaid program occurs with outpatient and clinical services (physicians' services). Each state can design its own Medicaid outpatient and physician reimbursement package.

Unlike the rather universal popularity of the Medicare program, Medicaid has since its inception been beset by critics from all sides. The principal criticism has focused on the problems of costs and eligibility in the program. As noted, the definition of "medical indigence" was, at the beginning, left to the individual states. But since certain states, like California and New York, provided rather liberal income limits for participants, the federal government, in the 1967 amendments to the Social Security Act, set an upper limit at one and one-third times the states' AFDC limit. (AFDC stands for aid to the aged, to the permanently and totally disabled, to the blind, and to the families of dependent children.) Accordingly, many were eliminated from the medically indigent ranks, especially in New York State.

Additionally, as might have been predicted, Medicaid has become, in some states, a political football. Certain states, for example, New York, have established a freeze on Medicaid payments until the end of a certain number of years and have set payment ceilings to be determined by the state, in contrast to open-ended Medicare cost reimbursement formulas.

If we step back and take a look at the situation, we can see that Medicaid problems are really part of the "welfare crisis" and were predictable. As a welfare program paid out of general taxes, it tends to share the stigma attached by most middle class Americans to all welfare programs, especially considering that the Medicaid program appears to be inordinately expensive.

Blue Cross

Blue Cross is a nongovernmental, nonprofit corporation that offers an insurance program that covers certain hospital services and pays benefits based on a contract between an individual plan and the Blue Cross insurance program in a particular area. Blue Shield is the same arrangement for the physician component; in other words, it is very similar to the Part B portion of the Medicare legislation. Blue Cross contracts vary substantially in reimbursement, but basically, for inpatient care, they are similar to Medicare. Reimbursement to hospitals by Blue Cross plans represents a major percentage of hospital revenues in this country.

Many of the Blue Cross plans in the country contract with groups of hospitals. Some of these contracts may pay a hospital's customary charges while others limit payments by reasonable cost formulas used under Medicare and Medicaid. The contract arrangement with hospitals is unlike that of other commercial carriers.

Unlike other private insurance companies, Blue Cross plans in most states must obtain the approval of the state insurance commissioner for any rate increases. This process differs from increasing reimbursement under Medicare and Medicaid, both of which are tied to hospital costs.

Blue Cross plans establish their premiums based on the average cost of actual or anticipated hospital care used by all their subscribers within a selected geographic area or a particular industry or company. The rate does not vary for different groups or subgroups of Blue Cross subscribers; for example it does not vary based on claims of experience, age, sex, or health status. This method is referred to as the community rating method. Insurance plans that do not use a community rating method may use an experience-rated scheme.

Self-Pay and Other Insurance

The fourth major type of reimbursement is used by those patients who pay their own individual hospital bills or have commercial insurance companies other than Blue Cross to cover their hospitalization. Though many insurance companies cover hospital services, they, unlike Blue Cross, do not contract directly with the hospitals. Reimbursement to the hospitals is generally made either through the patient, who then pays the hospital, or by assignment, in which case the patient "assigns" the reimbursement directly to the hospital. In both cases, patients are ultimately responsible for their bills. Generally, hospitals receive payment from such patients on a customary charge basis, not on a reasonable cost basis.

CONTRACTUAL ADJUSTMENTS

It is important to note that the hospital must account for its revenue as though it had received its full or customary charge, even though it knows it will not receive it from Medicare or Medicaid, or, in some instances, even from Blue Cross. The difference between the charge for the service and what is actually received from Medicare or Medicaid is termed a contractual adjustment; in retail businesses, it would be considered an allowance. This contractual adjustment must be shown as a deduction from gross revenues in the hospital's financial statements. Contractual adjustments are very similar to trade discounts that a retail business might give its customers in the private sector. The number of patients who pay their own way (self-pay patients) is declining each year. A recent study shows that less than 10 percent of hospital patients pay their own way: this is down from a 1967 figure of 12 percent. It thus becomes clear that the methods used by the third parties to assess "reasonable cost" will greatly affect the future of hospital reimbursement.[4]

HOSPITAL COSTS

Since 1966, with the start of Medicare, hospital costs have increased on average by 14 percent per year. Aside from the ordinary inflation felt by all sectors of our economy, the major factors contributing to this increase include the following:

- Medicare and Medicaid programs that reimburse hospitals costs

- major advances in technological equipment and treatment techniques

- greater use of inpatient services and the ancillary services

- dramatic increases in hospital personnel costs

The average hospital's salaries and wages and other employee benefits account for approximately two-thirds of the hospital's total operating cost. Since the average number of employees required for patient care has almost doubled since 1946, it becomes clear that much of the hospital's increased cost is in the area of personnel. Furthermore, it is more and more common for physicians to be employed directly by hospitals. Depending on the method of payment, the hospitals could be paying the salaries of these physicians, again adding to the increase in cost. Most industries have both fixed and variable costs. However, the hospital industry does not have the large variable cost that certain industries have. Therefore, while a normal business can react with layoffs and cutbacks or even shutdowns of the plant, it is difficult for a hospital to react on a timely basis to reductions in patient days or units of service.

HOSPITAL ACCOUNTING

Now that the hospital receives much of its reimbursement based on cost, it is necessary to keep accurate accounting records that describe the status and activities of the hospital. Accounting is the language of all business activities. Even though the hospital may be a nonprofit institution, it must adhere to strict accounting rules. The accounting records are, in the final analysis, the reports that express in dollars and cents the financial status of the hospital. Not all hospital accounting is uniform. However, with the passage of Medicare legislation in 1966, many hospitals now account for their activities in very similar ways. Indeed, the similarities between hospitals are much more apparent than their individual peculiarities.

Hospital accounting is commonly called "fund accounting." This kind of accounting was adopted by hospitals because they are the beneficiaries of many philanthropic efforts in the community. Since hospitals are the recipient of endowment funds and gifts for very special purposes, it is necessary for them to have more than one fund. Establishment of these individual funds places the hospital and its board in a fiduciary position that must adhere to the strict wishes of the donor. In order to carry out this responsibility, it has been necessary to separate endowment funds and gifts from other assets of the hospital. The American Institute of Certified Public Accountants (AICPA) now requires that such restricted resources be disclosed for external reporting purposes.[5]

In fund accounting, each distinct phase of financial activity is handled as a separate accounting entry with its own particular objective. Each of the separate funds, or accounts, is self-balancing (for an explanation of these accounts, see Appendix B). Fund accounting is a technique that accounts for separate entities in a single hospital or institution. Each separate fund represents a distinct phase of the hospital's financial obligations and operations. The hospital is legally responsible for a separate accounting of each of these funds.

Most nonprofit hospitals have four distinct funds or basic sets of books that are interrelated. These are the general fund, the plant fund, the endowment fund, and the special fund. For the employee and the community, the operations of the hospital appear to be reflected in the general fund. This fund has several categories, including assets; liabilities; net worth; gross income, which comes from reimbursements; allowances, such as contractual adjustments; net income; other income, which frequently comes from nonoperations, such as gift shops and interest income; total income expenses, a major component of which is salaries and wages, discussed earlier; and, finally, the net gain or loss for the accounting period. In summary, the hospital's operating fund is an account for the hospital's day-to-day financial activities that are not required to be accounted for in any separate or special fund or subcategory group. It is the most active fund in the hospital.

HILL-BURTON OBLIGATIONS

As mentioned in Chapter 2, in 1946 the federal government passed the Hospital Survey and Construction Act, called the Hill-Burton Program. This act allowed government funds to be used for the construction and renovation of hospitals. Many hospitals have been totally or partially funded by Hill-Burton monies, either by grants, loans, or other subsidies.

A hospital that has received any federal Hill-Burton assistance has a duty to:

1. provide a certain amount of free care to patients, and
2. provide a community service to its patients.

The most onerous of these two requirements is the free-care restriction. The free-care ruling stipulates that a hospital must provide uncompensated services in amounts equal to or exceeding either 3 percent of its operating costs for the preceding fiscal year or 10 percent of its federal assistance (i.e., Hill-Burton funds it has received), whichever is less. To carry out this obligation, hospitals must adopt a written plan for the distribution of free care, including public notice of the uncompensated services to be read by the public.

Financial and Statistical Reports

At the conclusion of a given accounting period (usually every month), the hospital issues certain internal financial statements. Individual hospitals will vary on the specific formats of these documents, but generally they include (1) a statement of revenue and expenses (or profit and loss) for the period, (2) a balance sheet, (3) a statement of changes in the balances of the various hospital funds, and (4) a statement of changes in the hospital's financial position. Hospitals also publish, along with these financial statements, statistical reports on the key hospital indicators. For example, admissions, patient days, and selected tests performed are compared with these in the last reporting period and in the previous year and possibly also with the hospital's budget of volume. A set of typical hospital financial statements, together with a list of financial and statistical definitions, is shown in Appendix B.

The Public Accounting Firm

It is the responsibility of hospital management and the controller to regularly generate internal financial statements, including the revenue and expense statement and the balance sheet. However, suppose the internal records and reports are inaccurate, and the reports do not accurately reflect the hospital's financial operations. How does a hospital board of trustees or the administrator determine the inaccuracies? Traditionally, hospitals have hired certified public accounting (CPA) firms to conduct annually an audit of the hospital's financial reports.

The auditing firm monitors the hospital's internal controls, verifies the values of the hospital's assets, and traces accounting transactions. In essence, the firm renders a "second opinion" on the hospital's financial matters. It generates its own annual financial reports, which are referred to as the certified statements. Most firms also issue a management letter that accompanies the financial reports. The management letter describes for the board and the administration those financial areas that require corrective action. In the era of heavy third party reimbursement, the auditors can aid hospitals that are seeking to maximize their reimbursements.

There are hundreds of certified public accounting firms in the United States that have experience in working with hospitals. They range in size from a one- or two-man operation to the very large international firms with vast staffs and numerous offices. Historically, the eight largest of these firms have been referred to as the "big eight." Employment of the auditing firm and receipts of their report are functions of the board of trustees.

COST CONTAINMENT

Hospital administrators, just as all Americans, are concerned with inflation and excessive costs. This concern has demonstrated itself in cost containment legislation. The federal government has been aggressive in seeking solutions to the inflationary health care issue, using its existing medical and health planning laws in cost containment efforts. The American Hospital Association has also initiated a voluntary effort to aid hospitals in containing costs. It is reasonable to assume that as inflation continues, Congress will continue to review cost containment legislation and other branches and departments of the government will continue their efforts to tighten regulations in the health care industry in an attempt to gain more control over hospital costs.

NOTES

1. Howard Berman and Lewis Weeks, *The Financial Management of Hospitals* (Ann Arbor, Mich.: Health Administration Press, 1976), p. 62.

2. Ibid., pp. 62-64.

3. U.S. Senate, Committee on Finance, *Medicare and Medicaid: Problems, Issues and Alternatives*, Report of the Staff to the Committee on Finance, 91st Cong., 1st sess., 1970, p. 1.

4. Merian Kirchner, "The Real World of Hospital Finance," *Medical Economics*, February 6, 1978, p. 219.

5. W. Glenn Cannon, Bernard O'Neil, Jr., and Allen Weltmann, *A Layman's Guide to Hospitals, An Introduction to Finance and Economics* (Coopers & Lybrand, 1978), p. 13.

Chapter 17

Business Functions

Key Terms

Controller ≈ *Accrual accounting* ≈ *Chart of accounts* ≈ *Posting entries* ≈ *Accounts receivable* ≈ *Cashier* ≈ *Hospital information system (HIS)* ≈ *"On-line" management reports*

INTRODUCTION

We have looked at two of the three major financial functions of the hospital. First, we have identified where and how the hospital receives its revenue. Second, we have analyzed how a hospital structures its operating, cash, and capital budgets. Now let us review the internal hospital business functions.

The hospital's functions and responsibilities in this area include (1) the maintenance of adequate accounting systems for all income and expenditures; (2) the development and coordination of the budget control mechanism; (3) credit and collections procedures; (4) collection of cash and banking procedures; (5) the maintenance of internal controls; (6) the compilation of pertinent departmental statistics in conjunction with the medical records department; and (7) the preparation of financial reports that can be invaluable tools for the administrator.

Organizationally, the individual responsible for these internal functions is either the controller or, in large institutions, the director of fiscal services. In either case, the individual reports directly to the CEO. A controller's responsibilities extend to all phases of financial management of the hospital, including general accounting and bookkeeping, patient accounts, and various aspects of financial reporting. Generally, under the controller is a business office manager and possibly a patient accounts manager, as well as a senior accountant (the individual in charge of the accounting division). The controller consults frequently with the hospital administrator and the numerous hospital department heads. The controller's knowledge of all phases of the hospital's finances provides a basis for recommending ways to improve the hospital's services. Recently, controllers have been emphasizing means of decreasing costs and improving third party reimbursement. Controllers are experts in analyzing data and inspecting reports. Through these accounting records, from which the financial statements are prepared, the hospital can determine whether it is financially sound or not.

ACCOUNTING RECORDS

The accounting records describe the financial status of the hospital. As the language of all business and economic activity, accounting is the tool that controls the hospital's economic transactions. Accounting is a way of classifying and interpreting the transactions, or groups of transactions, that occur in a hospital. A key criterion in adequate hospital accounting is uniformity. When Medicare legislation became effective in 1966, hospitals began to develop similar hospital accounts. However, there still exists important individual differences in hospital accounting.

It is not enough for the financial manager and hospital administrator to know that a certain department spent more than it received from its operations or that it spent more than its budget. The reason for the excess expenditure must be known so that it can be analyzed and administrative action taken to control the excessive use. Accounting is the discipline that permits adequate records to be maintained in order for management to take such action. Accounting provides an effective administrative device for reviewing the utilization of supplies and equipment, employee hours worked, and salaries paid.

Hospitals operate on an accrual basis of accounting. Under this system, income is recorded in the period in which it is received, as opposed to a cash basis, under which income is recorded when cash is received. Similarly, the accrual basis provides for the recording of expenses in the period in which they are incurred and for the recording of assets in the period in which they are acquired. In a cash basis method, the recording of expenses and asset acquisitions is made at the time the cash is disbursed for each item. It is important to understand these two approaches to accounting. The accrual basis method is more accurate and more complete. For hospitals, it is more productive than the cash basis method.

Depending on their accounting records and the order in which they are kept, hospitals usually follow the uniform classification of accounts shown in the American Hospital Association's *Chart of Accounts for Hospitals*. The hospital accountant is the principal person assigned the responsibility for the hospital's accounting system. The accountant must be familiar with current accounting procedures and statistical financial analyses used in the hospital field. The accountant works under the controller and also works closely with the business office manager and the data processing department. The senior accountant supervises the recording (posting) of entries in hospital ledgers and trial balances to ensure the accuracy of the records. Generally, the accountant completes any tax statements the hospital must submit and files cost reports with Medicare and other insurance plans.

THE BUSINESS OFFICE

The business office manager supervises an office of personnel and controls such functions as inpatient and outpatient billing, the cashiering functions, and the frequent credit and collection functions of the hospital. Keeping track of patients' bills, or the accounts receivable function, is crucial to the hospital, since it is through such billing that the hospital receives most of its income. This section of the business office maintains accurate billing records, checks the amounts received against patients' bills, compares them to hospital rates to ensure accuracy, and records the charges with the bookkeeping machine or through the data processing section. The accounts receivable section sends out itemized statements to the patients, showing payments received and any balance due. This section also adjusts the balances when payments are received from the hospital cashier.

The cashier plays a vital role in the public relations of the hospital, as well as in the collection of cash. Frequently, the cashier accepts deposits from patients who are admitted and receives cash or checks when patients are discharged. Frequently, the cashier must explain the hospital's billing forms and answer a variety of patient inquiries, as well as issue receipts for all transactions. The cashier must maintain very accurate transaction records. Cash received is balanced at the close of each day. The cashier may also store a patient's valuables or belongings (such as watches or jewelry) during the patient's stay in the hospital.

DATA PROCESSING

Though data processing is not limited to the business office or financial functions, it is discussed under internal financial operations since, at the beginning, the computer was limited largely to accounting, payroll, inventory, and other financial activities. It has thus become closely associated with the controller and with the financial functions of the hospital. The computer and data processing techniques are being used increasingly in master planning decisions with regard to medical records, administrative research, the laboratories, nursing activities, and other patient care activities.

The age of computers in the hospital field began around the mid-1950s, and the use of computers has since increased rapidly to include most hospitals in the country. Yet, though there has been great progress toward the use of a total hospital information system (HIS) and other applications, the state of the art still tends to be most sophisticated in the financial area. For this reason, hospitals usually have a separate data processing section or department under the guidance of the controller.

The director of the data processing section (sometimes called a manager or coordinator) provides for the function and coordination of all data processing activities within the institution. These data processing operations can be quite complex. It is the data processing manager's responsibility to interpret these operations and to educate the hospital department heads on the use of the computer.

When business functions are put into the computer, the statistics either are recorded at the department level and then brought up to the computer room for keypunching and input, or they can be inputted directly to the computer. The latter is referred to as being "on line." From these statistics and patient charges, the patients' bills are generated. As a byproduct, a host of important statistical and management reports are also developed. After the patient accounting system has been put into the computer, the rest of the accounting system of the hospital (starting with the hospital's general ledger) can also be put into the computer. Other financial related activities include the hospital payroll and the hospital's purchasing and inventory control system.

Data processing and the use of the computer alone are no panacea for the processing of hospital bills. They are no substitute for scientific management and are not necessarily a way to cut costs. Programming the computer can be expensive, and so can the hardware. However, there is no doubt that the accurate, timely, and rapid recordkeeping and reporting potential of the computer can be a tremendous help to hospital management in making financial decisions.

Every business has a financial side, and the hospital is no exception. The financial aspects of a hospital are the responsibility of the board of trustees. But, it is through the functions of the business office, the application of the budget, and the determination of rates that the board determines its fiscal policy.

Part VIII

Evaluating the Care

Chapter 18

Medical Records

Key Terms

Progress notes ~ Source-oriented medical record ~ Problem-oriented medical record ~ SOAP ~ Medical records administrator ~ Clinical Information System (CIS) ~ Discharge abstract ~ Microfilming ~ Delinquent medical records ~ Release of medical information ~ Privileged communication

INTRODUCTION

The hospital medical record has undergone great changes over the last two decades. These changes are due to the greater demand and use of the information contained in the medical record. The upsurge of interest in the medical record has been aided by the increase in the complexity of medical care and the renewed interest in the information carried in the medical record. This interest has been generated by a variety of growing parahealth professions that work within the hospital. Also, there are demands from third parties, including Medicare, PSRO, and other federal legislation, that have increased the need for access to the patient's medical record. Hospitals are required to conduct utilization reviews and medical audits that use the medical record. The computer, as a tool in the health information and management system, frequently interfaces with the patient's medical record. This has created a whole new discipline and scientific approach in dealing with the record. All of these factors have added to the growth and complexity of the hospital's medical records department.

183

PURPOSE OF THE MEDICAL RECORD

According to the American Hospital Association,

> the primary purpose of the medical record is to document the course of
> the patient's illness and treatment (medical care) during a particular
> period and during any subsequent period as an inpatient or outpatient.
> As such, it is an important tool in medical practice. It serves as a basis
> for the planning and evaluation of individual patient care and for the
> communication between the physician and other professionals con-
> tributing to the patient's care. The record's secondary purpose may be
> to 1) meet the legal requirements imposed on the hospital and the
> physician and 2) provide clinical data of interest to research systems.[1]

The JCAH states that the purposes of a hospital patient medical record are (1) to
provide a basis for planning the patient's care, (2) to furnish evidence that the
patient's medical evaluation and treatment were adequate during the hospital stay,
(3) to provide a communication vehicle between the health professionals contributing to the patient's care, (4) to supply the legal documents in the interest of
the patient, the hospital, and the health care practitioners, and (5) to provide a data
base for continuing education and research.[2]

DEFINITION OF A MEDICAL RECORD

The Commission on Medical Malpractice (sponsored by the Department of
Health, Education and Welfare) indicated in its very extensive 1973 report that
the hospital's medical record and the physician's office medical records are more
than a series of physician communications to other health professionals. The
commission pointed out that a medical record represents a

> complex communication between a health professional, including a
> written history and physical, progress notes, the nurses' notes, con-
> sultations, laboratory reports, operation summaries, discharge sum-
> maries, and the like. During the course of a particular hospitalization,
> the record may include a large spectrum of speculation and observation
> as the various members of the health team contribute thoughts and
> observations that lead eventually to the final diagnosis.[3]

TRADITIONAL MEDICAL RECORDS

Historically, medical records have been a chronological assembly of notes, forms, reports, and summaries. The traditional or classical record, used in most hospitals today, is a combination of these forms, reports, and notes. The forms are the vehicle for the physician and health practitioners to record the patient's illness and course of recovery. Reports (based on studies such as laboratory tests, x-ray examinations, and operating room procedures) are also included in the medical record. Usually, the record contains written notations, clinical analyses, and handwritten or typed consultation summaries. All of these forms and reports are usually contained in a folder called a chart. Most often the record is maintained in chronological order; that is, the first events regarding the patient in the hospital are noted first in the medical record, followed by subsequent occurrences.

Thus, the traditional record is a package of forms and reports, including the patient's admission form, medical history, physical examination form, and laboratory, x-ray and special report forms. If the patient undergoes surgery, there will usually be authorization and consent forms (including a signed authorization or informed consent) obtained prior to surgery. The patient's anesthesia record will usually be attached to the surgeon's operative report, which is usually dictated and typed. Frequently, physicians' orders will follow the admission form. These orders are on forms, maintained in chronological fashion, by which the physician communicates to the nurses and other health care professionals instructions for carrying out the patient's diagnosis and therapy. Usually near the physician's order sheets are progress note sheets. The progress note sheets are often the largest part of any patient's medical record. The nurses' notes or nursing records are really progress notes from a nursing standpoint. The nursing notes contain the nurses' around-the-clock observations of the patient. Finally, in the record there will be a discharge order written on the physician's order blank, indicating that the patient can be discharged. Following the discharge of the patient, it is required that the physician dictate a narrative summary; this is usually typed and placed into the medical record after the patient has left the hospital. Although this is the last document recorded by the physician, it is generally placed in first position when the record is finally stored so that reviewers can quickly see the course of the patient's hospital stay.

The arrangement and dictating of all these separate forms in chronological order is the traditional or classical method of maintaining hospital patient medical records. More recently, the traditional record has become known as the source-oriented medical record. Prior to the permanent filing of the medical record in storage, the traditional record is somewhat rearranged as follows: The demographic data and identification data come first, followed by the patient's historical medical information and base line medical data; finally nursing data and nursing notes are stored in the record.

THE PROBLEM-ORIENTED MEDICAL RECORD

For years, the traditional or classical medical record was the only model available to hospitals and physicians. However, in 1960, Dr. Lawrence Weed of the University of Vermont Medical School initiated a new way of recording a patient's medical problems. He devised a problem-oriented medical record or POMR. As the name implies, Weed's system highlights the patient's problems rather than bury them chronologically as the classical medical record does. The POMR is supposed to aid the physician by identifying the patient's problems and then outlining the plan for a course of treatment for the specified problems. The emphasis in the POMR is to coordinate the various health skills, and is not limited to only those of the physician. The emphasis is on solving the patient's whole problem, not just episodic situations. The POMR has been reported to be a better organized, more rational, and more consistent way of gathering medical facts about the patient's clinical problems. It provides an organized way of planning the therapy and following the patient's progress. Compared with the traditional record, the advantages of POMR become evident. Apart from the fact that the POMR tends to be easier for medical students and for health professionals to use, it has these additional advantages:

- It is easier to use as an educational tool.

- It is a more logical system for PSRO and other agencies to review.

- It lends itself better to a rational review of medical progress and care rendered.

- It allows for improved continuity of care, since the professionals all use the same set of recording rules (the patient's problems are thereby not lost or as easily confused).

- It is more adaptable to computerization.

- It is easier for the nonmedical personnel to read.

In the traditional medical record, chronological events, specific forms, and reports are the basis of the record. The POMR system uses specific elements, namely, data base information that is gathered together and clearly recorded, and a numbered list of specific patient problems. In the POMR system, a problem-oriented plan is agreed upon and as in the traditional system, progress notes made. But, in the POMR, these notes refer specifically to the numbered patient problems. In recording POMR progress notes, a definite system called "SOAP" is used, incorporating (1) *s*ubjective data, (2) *o*bjective data, (3) *a*ssessment or interpretation of impressions, and (4) an ongoing clinical *p*lan for the patient.

THE MEDICAL RECORDS DEPARTMENT

Medical records have been retained for hundreds of years. Even before pencil and paper, we can assume that some of the hieroglyphics on Egyptian tombs and temples referred to medical aspects of the deceased. A new impetus in medical records departments and medical records administration was launched early in the 1900s. In 1912, interested medical record librarians gathered at the Massachusetts General Hospital to discuss their common interests. In 1928, the Association of Record Librarians of North America was born. This later became known as the American Association of Medical Records Librarians. Today the JCAH requires that "the Medical Record Department shall be provided with adequate direction, staffing and facilities to perform all required functions."[4] This means that a "qualified medical record individual, responsible to the Chief Executive Officer or his designee, shall be employed on at least a part-time basis consistent with the needs of the hospital medical staff. This individual shall be either a Registered Record Administrator or Accredited Record Technician based on successful completion of examination requirements of the American Medical Record Association."[5]

Part of the medical record administrator's job is to organize and manage the medical record system and to provide efficient medical record services to the hospital. Specifically, this person's duties include: (1) planning, designing, and technically evaluating patient information; (2) planning, directing, and controlling the administration of the medical record department and its services; (3) aiding the medical staff in its work on medical records; (4) developing statistical reports for management and the medical staff; and (5) analyzing technical evaluations of health records and indices.[6]

Hospital medical records are highly visible instruments used in the evaluation of patient care. This being the case, it is very common for third parties, and especially the JCAH, during their annual or biannual surveys to study and review carefully the patients' medical records.

One of the traditional areas that is almost always reviewed is the timely completion of the medical record. Outside reviewers can be expected to inspect the matter of delinquent medical records at any given point in time during the survey. In fact, if the delinquent record problems are serious, they could jeopardize the hospital's accreditation by the JCAH.

Yet, though the medical record presents a wealth of data for countless third parties, quality assurance reviewers, and third party payers, one of the most common problems in medical records still remains that of delinquent medical records. Many physicians do not complete their medical records in a timely and accurate manner. This tends to be a chronic problem faced by medical record administrators across the country. In the final analysis, the most potent weapon against these delinquencies is suspension of privileges of physicians until they complete their records.

Medical records administrators are constantly attempting to make the processing of medical records and information more efficient. One area that shows promise for increased efficiency in the storage and handling of information is the word processing computer. Usually this type of computer hardware is used in conjunction with a centralized medical typing pool. With the ease and speed permitted by the word processing computer, handwritten records can be replaced by typed reports, including patient histories, results of physical examinations, and consultant reports.

Many hospitals participate in a shared computer medical record system called the Professional Activity Study (PAS). The PAS is purchased from the Commission on Professional Hospital Activities (CPHA), a nonprofit computer center, located in Ann Arbor, Michigan. With this system, the hospital's medical records technicians complete a discharge abstract for every discharged patient. The information on the abstract is then displayed and returned to the hospital in the form of a series of monthly and semiannual reports showing such data as the patient's average length of stay by disease categories and the number of clinical tests and studies performed during the period. An extension of the PAS that displays hospital clinical data quarterly is called the Medical Audit Program (MAP). MAP reports are used in continuous, comprehensive medical audits and retrospective utilization reviews.

ORGANIZATION OF THE DEPARTMENT

The organization and staffing of the medical record department reflect in a very straightforward manner the tasks and functions of the department. The department is staffed to handle (1) release of information, (2) admission and discharge analyses, (3) medical transcriptions, (4) coding and abstracting (generally this involves diagnostic and procedural coding), and (5) storage and retrieval.

In the area of statistics and recordkeeping, the statistical section of the medical records department provides the input to many of the computerized data services that hospitals use to generate computerized patient data profiles. The primary source of these data is the patient's discharge abstract that is submitted to computerized agencies, such as the Hospital Utilization Program (HUP) or the Commission on Professional Hospital Activities (CPHA). These data are summarized in computer language and sent to a computer with large memory banks. The hospitals can then receive the information in a readable and quickly retrievable fashion.

Typically, a medical record is hard copy; that is, it is bound in paper. However, as bulk storage becomes a problem and space becomes more scarce, the microfilming of medical records has become quite common. In recent years, microfilm formats have improved greatly. Earlier, rolls of film were put into cartridges and could be indexed. Today, motor viewers used for high speed retrieval have been replaced in some areas by microfiche, which is a more efficient, cost effective means of storage and retrieval.

The transcription section of the medical record department is an area in which medical typists transcribe the summaries and reports dictated by physicians onto paper for filing in the medical record. At one time, many hospitals employed medical transcribers; today, it is common to use outside transcription services. With these outside systems, the transcription is dictated over the telephone, typed, and then sent by messenger or mail to the hospital. This system offers the hospital the advantage of not having to deal with various hospital employees. Also, the hospital is paying exactly for what it receives in typing, and the outside service relieves the hospital from the task of maintaining a bank of technical transcription equipment.

THE MEDICAL RECORDS COMMITTEE

The medical staff's medical records committee is the liaison between the medical record department and the physicians in the hospital. This committee is charged with the responsibility of reviewing and evaluating the medical records function. These tasks should be performed not less than quarterly. Generally, based on random sampling and recommendations from a variety of medical sources, the committee will review certain records on a regular basis for appropriateness. However, the principal responsibility for quality of peer review rests with the medical staff's audit and utilization review committees.

The medical records committee's principal responsibility is to supervise the organization of the record. The committee must review and approve all new medical record forms. In view of the fact that the traditional record is a potpourri of medical forms, this can be, at certain hospitals, a very time-consuming task. The committee should evaluate the accuracy of certain record notations relating to management and administrative matters of the record. For example, if physicians are not writing the discharge diagnosis on the medical record at the proper time or in the proper place, the medical records committee should take directive action. It is the committee's responsibility to police the traditional and chronic problem of physicians' delinquency in completing medical records.

The medical records committee does not generally get involved in making recommendations on management issues in the medical records department. For example, filing procedures, coding of medical records, storage, microfilming potentials, and preservation of certain sections of the record are matters usually left to the medical records administrator in conjunction with the hospital management.

However, if the hospital were to change from a traditional medical record system to a problem-oriented medical record system, this committee would play a key role in analyzing the pro's and con's of switching.

LEGAL REQUIREMENTS

The medical records administrator is the custodian of the medical records and must be alert to certain legal requirements with regard to the handling and release of medical information and medical records. The maintenance of medical records is governed by the Uniform Business Record Evidence Act. Accordingly, the records are retained as part of the day-to-day business of the hospital.

Rules on the release of medical information vary from state to state. Thus, the medical records administrator must understand the specific rules in the state in which the hospital is located. The medical records administrator is also expected to handle privileged communications with individuals, through the courts or various governmental agencies under established hospital policy, and to follow state and federal rules and laws. The medical records administrator is the special guardian of medical records that are in litigation (for example, malpractice suits). In that capacity, the administrator has to testify (orally or in writing) at legal hearings and sometimes actually has to go to court to indicate that the hospital medical record is the accurate document it is purported to be.

COMPUTERIZED MEDICAL RECORDS

Before 1960, electronic computers were sparsely used in hospitals. Those in use were primarily self-contained within functional areas, such as admissions or the patient accounting departments. There were, however, mechanical aids for data processing, such as mechanical bookkeeping machines and punched card equipment. As the hospitals moved into the 1960s, computers became a larger factor in the management of information. As we have noted, a heavy emphasis was placed on business functions, with some excellent computerized packages used for all accounting functions. However, there was very little application of computers to clinical information or the medical information system. With the upsurge in the use of computers in the 1960s, many hospitals experienced serious problems as a result of rushing into computerized information systems before they really understood what the capabilities were or how the systems worked.

As computer technology moved into the 1970s, however, two important advances had an impact on hospitals: (1) Many computers offered ''on-line'' systems that were able to provide the hospital staff with direct access to computerized data bases through decentralized communications terminals. (2) The development of the relatively inexpensive minicomputer market allowed hospitals to bundle their systems and, through the use of minicomputers, to integrate subsystems into one overall system.

In the area of computerized medical record information, the Clinical Information System (CIS) involved "the organized processing, storage, and retrieval of information to support patient care activities in the hospital. Specific CIS and computer applications may be categorized as follows: computer-aided diagnosis; computer-aided treatment and follow-up; patient monitoring systems; laboratory automation; medical records indexing and retrieval; pharmacy information systems."[7]

Applications of the CIS have been developed for both the traditional and problem-oriented medical record. One such system that has been in operation for several years in the Massachusetts General Hospital in Boston is called MUMPS (Massachusetts General Hospital Utility-Programing System). Applications of MUMPS have been developed in the following areas: laboratory test reporting, automated patient histories, patient summary reports, critical patient care planning, medical education, medical examination, automated medication systems, physician-generated narrative notes, statistical packages, and medical care utilization statistics. Given the kinds of material that have to be computerized, medical information systems are very complex to develop and to maintain, since it is necessary to allow multiple inputs and inquiries and to have a large capacity of peripheral storage. One of the most important aspects of developing information systems is getting user acceptance, that is, making it comfortable for nurses, physicians, and other health care professionals to use sophisticated computerized systems.

The implementation of computerized medical information systems is in its infancy. It is clear, however, that when such systems become more widely available and used, they will be a powerful force for change in the traditional hospital environment. Such traditional situations as staffing patterns and interpersonal relationships, for example, physicians' and nurses' roles, will have to adjust to the new computer technology. The fastest avenue to acceptance may lie with the computerized problem-oriented medical record, since, compared to the traditional record, it is more organized, and the ground rules for using it are more easily understood.

NOTES

1. American Hospital Association, *Hospital Medical Records—Guidelines for Their Use and the Release of Medical Information* (Chicago, Ill.: 1972), p. 3.

2. Joint Commission on Accreditation of Hospitals, *Accreditation Manual for Hospitals—1980 Edition* (Chicago, Ill.: JCAH, 1979), p. 83.

3. Department of Health, Education and Welfare, *Report of the Secretary's Commission on Medical Malpractice,* DHEW Publication no. (05)73-88, 1972, p. 76.

4. Joint Commission, *Accreditation Manual,* p. 90.

5. Ibid., p. 90.

6. American Hospital Association, *Medical Record Departments in Hospitals: Guide to Organization* (Chicago, Ill.: American Hospital Association, 1972), p. 3.

7. Charles T. Austin and Barry R. Greene, "Hospital Information Systems: A Current Perspective," *Inquiry,* June 1978, p. 96.

Chapter 19

Quality Assurance

American College of Surgeons ≈ Professional Standards Review Organization (PSRO) ≈ Committee structure of the medical staff ≈ Autopsies ≈ Credentials committee ≈ Tissue committee ≈ Quality Assurance Program (QAP) ≈ Utilization review (UR) committee ≈ Medical audit (MA) committee ≈ Structure ≈ Process ≈ Outcome ≈ Retrospective review ≈ Darling case

DEFINITION

The "quality" part of quality assurance is not easy to define. To define it we must use terms like characteristic, property, and attribute—all of them as difficult to define as quality itself. One approach is to look at a few things that quality is not. In medicine it is not the same as quantity. Nor is it the same as cost, cost efficiency, utilization of health care, or medical care. Quality is not consistent across the board; it may vary from time to time in hospitals and among physicians. Finally, quality can denote either good or bad, and bad quality is as difficult to define as good quality.

Having stated all of this, what then is quality? A traditional view of physicians is that quality of health care must depend upon the credentials of the provider. There is a belief that the physicians who are highly trained are probably better than those who are less well trained. Many believe that the real test of quality of care is: How did it turn out? To put it another way, when the physician and the medical team treated the patient, did the patient recover; and did the patient have good results?

Quality, according to some experts, is a function of the medical service given patients at a specific point in time by a specific doctor to a specific patient. You cannot evaluate after the fact adequately if you were not there rendering the care. The American Society of Internal Medicine and its committee on quality evaluation have defined quality as follows: "Quality medical care embodies a scientific approach to the establishment of a diagnosis and institution of appropriate therapy and management, designed to satisfy the overall needs of the patient. It should be readily available, efficiently rendered and properly documented."[1]

Quality assurance in hospitals is really an ongoing process. Its goals are to measure and to evaluate the professional services rendered to the patient in the hospital. Service in a proper quality assurance program is measured against a prevailing and accepted standard of professional care. The end product of quality assurance is the improvement of care; it is supposed to change the behavior of physicians and health team members and thereby improve the quality of care.

HISTORICAL REVIEW

There are records on the quality of care that go back as far as the eleventh century B.C., when Egyptian physicians were reported to be regulated by a certain law as to the nature and extent of their practice.[2] Quality assurance programs in America became common and were better understood following the early 1900s when Abraham Flexner presented his classic report on the quality of medical education in this country. In 1918, the American College of Surgeons initiated the Hospital Standardization Program to encourage uniform medical record formats and to facilitate accurate recording of the patient's medical course. In 1951, based on this effort, the JCAH was established. In the 1950s, the JCAH attempted to implement certain crude auditing procedures, but they did not prove to be very useful. It was left to the late 1960s and early 1970s for these methodologies to be refined. Meanwhile, for three decades, from the 1930s to the 1960s, the nation continued to debate the issue of national health insurance. Finally, with Public Law 89-97 in 1966, the Medicare and Medicaid programs became effective. This law gave birth to the concept that health care was a right of all of the people. With this law, the federal government became the largest purchaser or payer for health services in the nation.

Titles XVII and XIX of the Medicare program mandated hospitals to perform utilization review functions. Utilization review is the process designed to monitor the need for patient admission to the hospital and for the continued stay of each inpatient. Partly as an attempt to control spiraling health care costs, Congress in 1972 passed a Social Security amendment called Public Law 92-603. This legislation mandated Professional Standards Review Organizations (PSRO). Its champion was Senator Wallace Bennett, a Republican from Utah. In Senator Bennett's view,

> with respect to the quality, the suitability and the necessity of medical care, only doctors are qualified to pass judgment. We should not leave to the insurance companies or any hired administrators the task of

evaluating quality of medical care given to Medicare and Medicaid recipients. The converse of that, of course, is that doctors would like to have an opportunity to demonstrate that doctors themselves can avoid keeping people in hospitals too long—ordering unnecessary treatments, etc. So we developed the PSRO concept which envisions that the Secretary of HEW invite applications from groups of doctors who will accept as a profession the responsibility for reviewing the work of themselves and their peers in the area.[3]

With the PSRO legislation, a nationwide network of locally based physician groups was created to review the necessity, the quality, and the appropriateness of hospital care provided under the provisions of the Social Security Act. In short, PSROs are official organizations with authority mandated by the federal government to monitor the process of utilization review for federally funded patients and to monitor medical care evaluations (medical audits) performed by hospitals.

CLASSICAL TECHNIQUES

Before the advent of sophisticated PSRO programs, medical audits, utilization reviews, and medical care evaluation studies, the hospital used traditional quality control mechanisms, primarily through its committee structure of the medical staff organization. These traditional or classic control mechanisms stemmed from medical staff bylaws, rules, and regulations and drew their authority from the board of trustees. Even today, these control mechanisms are reviewed closely by JCAH surveyors and other third party inspectors.

Among the major quality control mechanisms that should be in each medical staff's bylaws is the committee structure. For example, the medical staff organization should have a medical records committee to review the contents, appropriateness, and timeliness of medical records. Another important quality control mechanism, though becoming less frequently used, is the procedure of conducting autopsies on deceased patients. Autopsies have dropped off precipitously in the last several years, due primarily to the phobia about malpractice that has hit the profession.

The credentials committee is charged with the responsibility of interviewing and reviewing the credentials and delineation of privileges for each new medical staff candidate. Also, every year or two, the committee reviews the members of the medical staff for appointments to the hospital. The tissue committee is another important committee that exercises control over quality. It is charged with the responsibility of studying and examining the tissue removed from surgical procedures; it renders its reports to the executive committee of the medical staff. Finally, the medical record department compiles statistical data highlighting such things as the number of admissions, the number of deaths in the hospital, the number of complications through infection control, and the like. Taken in the aggregate, the committee structure is the front line of quality assurance for the hospital. This, together with the JCAH standards survey that is conducted annually at least every two years, provides the hospital with a good first line of defense against poor quality.

NEWER APPROACHES

In 1971, the American Hospital Association (AHA) started to work on a "Quality Assurance Program for Medical Care in the Hospital" (QAP). The work and interest of the American Hospital Association in this area even predates PSRO, which gave additional impetus to hospitals to spend more time and attention on evaluating the quality rendered within its walls. In the 1970s, the QAP sponsored by the AHA was the principal framework used to monitor quality assurance in hospitals. The QAP envisioned two working committees: a utilization review committee (UR) and a medical audit committee (MA). The utilization review committee had five separate elements: (1) the certification of admission, (2) pre-admission testing, (3) length of stay (LOS) certification, (4) length of stay review, and (5) discharge planning. The medical audit phase of the program stressed the development of objective criteria and provided for detailed medical audits to be processed and measured against those criteria. The purpose of these two committees was to change physician behavior based on suggested courses of action identified in the UR and MA processes. The procedure included an educational process following the action of the two committees and, specifically, an educational effort to change physicians' behavior based on the results of the medical audit.

The JCAH has recently issued a new set of quality assurance standards for hospitals that will affect accreditation decisions in 1981. These new standards will replace the standards of the 1970s, which focused on the mechanics of the medical audit process in a "cookbook"-like fashion. According to the JCAH, the standards were revised because the previous ones were ineffective, created inefficiencies in hospital committees and activities, and provided an overemphasis on patient care audit and utilization review. The commission also recognized that there were other influences that affect quality, such as cost containment and legal cases. The new standards require each hospital to design a quality assurance strategy based on its own needs and resources. Essentially, the JCAH is seeking to streamline the committee structure. Balancing continued use of the medical audit and the importance of all quality assurance activities, including an emphasis on risk management activities, are emphasized.

DEFINING AUDIT TERMS

The medical audit is one of the principal tools used to evaluate quality care in institutions. It is therefore necessary to understand clearly certain definitions used in the medical audit process. There are three generally accepted systems used in conducting a medical audit: the structure system, the process system, and the outcome system.

The structure system is one in which the hospital and its medical staff evaluate the setting in which care is rendered and resources made available to the physician and practitioner to give the care; this system deals primarily with the adequacy of the hospital's facilities and manpower. Process audit refers to what the physician actually does to diagnose and to treat the patient; this involves the source of medical care and the patient's compliance with the physician's orders. Outcome audit concerns the actual results of the care given. For example, did the patient respond properly to treatment? What was the mortality rate for treatment? Was the patient able to perform regular daily activities? And did the patient have any psychological effects?

Because there are three kinds of structures or systems for evaluation, the hospital has the opportunity to review quality while the patient is in the hospital and also retrospectively in terms of what happened after the patient left the hospital, based on the medical record. Traditional medical audits in the hospital usually included retrospective review of the medical care process, based on the patient's medical record. More recently, the questions of outcome and patient satisfaction are also being considered.

Although the principal function of a medical audit should be to improve patient care, there are also byproducts. Deficiencies are noted and can be corrected. The audit method encourages coordination of physicians with other health team members in the planning of patient care. The documentation of patient care is improved through medical records. Additional direction is given to continuing education programs for physicians and health care personnel. The need for new equipment or facilities can be brought to the attention of the management of the hospital. Finally, a proper medical audit provides to the board of trustees written documentation of the status of the medical care as practiced in certain diagnoses in the hospital.

THE BOARD'S RESPONSIBILITY

In the 1965 landmark legal suit in the state of Illinois, *Darling v. Charleston Community Hospital,* the court ruled that a hospital and its board of trustees must assume shared responsibility for the medical care of the patients in the hospital.[4] Other court interpretations since then have confirmed the hospital's obligation to oversee the medical staff in the quality of care. The board of trustees should play a role in the hospital's structuring of quality control systems. It must make sure that the medical staff is well organized and that appropriate and effective medical audit procedures are implemented in the hospital.

THE STATE OF THE ART

Though reams of material have been written on the subject, the definition of quality is still an elusive one in the medical profession. One of the reasons is that it is very difficult to measure the process of caring for a patient and all the interpersonal and psychological aspects of that care, especially the relationship between the patient and physician. Many would agree with the statement of Walter J. McNerney, president of Blue Cross of America, that we do not have enough experience in quality assurance from an operational prospective and that the existing systems leave much to be desired.[5]

The PRSO program's main emphasis to date has been on the quantity of care as a cost saving measure rather than on quality assurance. There has been very little emphasis on ambulatory care and the evaluation of quality in the ambulatory part of the outcare picture. The role of the consumers has been a very passive one in quality assurance, notwithstanding the fact that the health systems agencies are supposed to be consumer-dominated. Thus, consumers have had very little impact on the medical audit and the utilization review processes.

In one observer's view, "quality assurance is the end result of effective management practices being applied to all areas of our health care system."[6] The author's observation is that, though quality assurance attempts have been with us for many years, the state of the art is relatively still in its infancy and has still to undergo a great deal of evolution. The record shows that the decade of the 1970s was a period of sorting out methodologies, particularly with regard to the medical audit. In the 1980s, with the new quality assurance standard instituted by the JCAH, hospitals seeking JCAH accreditation must coordinate or integrate as much as possible all quality assessment activities within a comprehensive, hospital-wide quality assurance program. The hope is that quality care requirements will be linked throughout the hospital. It is recognized that quality assessment techniques are dynamic in nature and are continually changing to keep up with the state of the art. The commission has attempted to be flexible in accommodating these changes and has accordingly designed its new standards to be flexible enough so that they can be implemented and administered effectively. There is reason to believe that the JCAH will continue to tailor its standards, change its methods, and evolve its quality assurance programs.

NOTES

1. W. Felch, "Practice Problems: The Assessment of Quality," *Internist,* December 1969, p. 20.
2. C. Buck, "Terms and Trends in Quality Assurance," *Trustee,* September 1975, p. 32.
3. "Peer Review, Is It Working?," *Review* 9, no. 1 (February 1976).
4. Darling v. Charleston Community Hospital, 211 N.E. 2d 253 (1965) cert. denied 383 V.S. 946 (1966).
5. Walter J. McNerney, "The Quandary of Quality Assessment," *New England Journal of Medicine* 295 (1976): 1505-1511.
6. Harold R. McAlindon, "Quality Assurance: The Management Role," *Administrative Brief, American College of Hospital Administrators,* July 1975, p. 1.

Chapter 20

Malpractice

Key Terms

Plaintiff ∿ *Captive insurance companies* ∿ *Defensive medicine* ∿ *Nork case* ∿
Medical malpractice

INTRODUCTION

The phenomenon of malpractice that began to flourish in the early 1960s has
continued to mushroom in the health care field. In one view, "medical malpractice
is a failure on the part of the provider of health care to conform to accepted
standards of skill and care or other misconduct which causes injury to a patient."[1]
In 1973, medical malpractice was defined in a very complete study by the
Department of Health, Education and Welfare. In the department's *Report of the
Secretary's Commission on Malpractice,* the following was stated:

> Medical malpractice has been defined as an injury to a patient caused by
> a health care provider's negligence; a malpractice claim is an allegation
> with or without foundation that an injury was caused by negligence;
> injury implies either physical or mental harm that occurs in the course
> of medical care whether or not it is caused by negligence; compensation
> requires proof of both an injury and a professional negligence.[2]

To win a malpractice suit, the plaintiff (the individual suing the hospital) must
meet two standards: First, the plaintiff must prove that the poor or unfortunate
results that occurred from the alleged malpractice were really negligence, not
solely a misadventure. Second, the plaintiff must prove that, because of the
unfortunate medical results, there resulted a financial loss or other damages from
the negligence.

SIZE OF THE PROBLEM

How big a problem is malpractice? It is impossible to determine the number of medical malpractice claims at any time. However, recent studies have indicated that medical malpractice claims have possibly tripled since 1970.[3] Not only has the incidence of malpractice suits increased dramatically, but the size of the average medical malpractice award has doubled over a recent six-year period.[4] In 1976, the average malpractice award was $27,708, almost twice the average award in 1970. It is interesting to note that this increase was twice the rate of increase in the general inflation index.[5] Today, very large awards are still with us in this country. For example, in Massachusetts a case was settled for 4.5 million dollars, and in California there have been awards of 4.0 million and 7.6 million dollars.[6] There is another case in California that may ultimately approach 14.0 million dollars.[7] Statistics from the National Association for Insurance Commissioners indicate that, on average, the plaintiffs in malpractices cases really do not benefit. In two-thirds of the cases studied by the association, the plaintiffs received nothing. Another 15 percent of the plaintiffs received less than $3,000 in settlement.[8]

WHO IS BEING SUED?

The HEW Secretary's Commission Report noted above listed the types of physicians most likely to be sued: surgeons, especially orthopedists, followed by anesthesiologists. According to a 1970 study, the percentage of malpractice claims by type of treatment were as follows: 57.2 percent surgical, 20.5 percent medical, 6.1 percent radiology, 1.6 percent pathology, and 14.6 percent all other treatments, including those in emergency rooms.[9] In the 1976 HEW Secretary's Commission review of malpractice, neurosurgeons, orthopedists, and plastic surgeons were the most frequent targets of malpractice claims. The fewest number of claims were targeted against the specialties of internal medicine, ophthalmology, and urology.[10] The same review indicated that surgical errors were mentioned in 33 percent of the malpractice claims while institutional (hospital) errors were cited in 32 percent of the claims. In the claims where injuries involved hospitals, 42 percent were likely to have occurred in the operating room, while 24 percent took place in the patient's room.[11] The irony in this mushrooming malpractice phenomenon is that apparently the standards of medicine in the United States have been rising during this period. Therefore, most experts agree that the rise in malpractice claims is not directly related to the quality of medical care provided. Perhaps higher medical bills have been a factor in the increase in suits. Or perhaps there have been more dramatic surgical procedures that were not a factor earlier. Or, finally, perhaps the public is taking abusive license on doctors and have become suit happy. Indeed, the lawyers themselves are not free from being sued for malpractice; and, in other areas, product liability insurance rates for manufacturers have skyrocketed.

INSURANCE COSTS

With the increase in malpractice suits over the last decade, many insurance companies will no longer insure health care professionals (physicians and hospitals). This has forced providers to form their own insurance pools or captive insurance companies. In many states, insurance companies are reluctant to write malpractice insurance policies because they are unable to forecast adequately the insurance costs in relation to the rate of inflation, the increasing number of malpractice suits brought to litigation, the skyrocketing award amounts, or their ability to justify the premium increases quickly enough to recapture losses. Also, a key factor in insurance companies leaving the market is their difficulty of managing insurance reserves in a period of unforeseen inflation coupled with investment uncertainty. The bottom line for the insurance companies is that they believe that the malpractice risks outweigh the potential returns. Perhaps the main reason insurance companies are uncertain about their investment is the length of time between the malpractice occurrence and the final resolution of the malpractice suit; this could be many years.

For the insurance companies who have remained in the malpractice field, there has been a staggering increase in premiums. For example, in New York State, in 1974, there was a request for a 200 percent increase after a 100 percent increase only six months previously. In another case, in 1975 in northern California, there was a 300 percent increase request. In Ohio, there was an increase request of 747 percent. Currently, some insurance companies are increasing their malpractice premiums by 200 to 600 percent.

DEFENSIVE MEDICINE

As a direct result of the medical malpractice crisis, there has been an alarming increase in defensive medicine practiced by physicians. In 1973 the HEW Secretary's Commission defined defensive medicine as "the alteration of modes of medical practice, induced by the threat of liability for the principal purpose of forestalling the possibility of law suits by patients as well as providing a good legal defense in the event such law suits are instituted."[12] The costs for the additional tests performed to protect the physician are staggering. The actual cost is not known, but estimates of the cost of defensive medicine range from between 3 to 7 billion dollars each year.[13] The practice of defensive medicine is widespread among physicians. In 1977, an American Medical Association poll revealed that 75 percent of the physicians included in the poll said they now practice defensive medicine.[14]

HOSPITAL LIABILITY FOR PHYSICIANS' ACTS

It is important to recognize that in some cases a hospital may be held liable for physicians' negligent acts. The most frequent occasion for this is when the hospital permits an incompetent physician to treat a patient. The hospital can be held liable even when the physician is not employed by the hospital. The institution is not held liable for the negligent act that caused harm to the patient, but it is held liable for its own negligence in permitting the physician to treat the patient. It is reasoned that a physician's incompetence should be known to hospital authorities.

One of the best known legal cases supporting this principle is *Gonzales v. Nork and Mercy Hospitals of Sacramento*. Similarly, a hospital can be held liable for failure to properly supervise the clinical privileges of a physician. The court's position on this principle is clear in *Darling vs. Charleston Community Memorial Hospital*. Ever since the Darling case the courts have imposed legal liabilities upon hospital boards and management for the supervision of clinical practices within an institution. In essence, the courts are saying that by appointing a physician to the medical staff, the hospital is guaranteeing that physician's competence. Accordingly, preventing malpractice claims and legal litigation is a joint effort among the hospital board, the medical staff, and hospital management.

ROLE OF THE MEDICAL RECORD

It may be two or three years after an incident occurred before a hospital administrator or physician receives a notice of suit. The next step is for the physician or the administrator to ask for the patient's medical record. The hospital medical record should depict in written fashion the course of the patient's care and treatment while in the hospital. The record provides the medium of communication among the members of the hospital health team. It is also frequently a factor in whether a plaintiff wins the case. Juries and malpractice lawyers are not likely to accept the reasoning that the chart was not written clearly enough at the time. The medical record must accurately reflect the true events of the hospitalization; there is no substitute for such documentation in winning a malpractice case.

When an administrator receives a suit against the hospital, frequently the physician is named also. It is a good procedure to make a copy of the medical record for the hospital's attorney as well as for the physician's attorney. The original medical record should be placed under lock and key in the medical record department while the case is in litigation.

NOTES

1. Charles A. Hoffman, "Dissenting Statement," *Report of the Secretary's Commission on Medical Malpractice,* DHEW publication no. (08) 73-88, 1973, p. 115.

2. U.S., Department of Health, Education and Welfare, 1973, *Report of the Secretary's Commission on Medical Malpractice,* DHEW publication no. (08) 73-88, p. 4.

3. Ann Landers, *The Ann Landers Encyclopedia A to Z* (New York, N.Y.: Ballantine Books, 1978), p. 701.

4. Risk Management, Crain News Service, "Malpractice Awards Double in Size," *Modern Health Care,* May 1979, p. 34.

5. Ibid.

6. "Malpractice—Increasing or Decreasing?" "Phico Info," *Bulletin No. 22,* November 14, 1978, p. 1.

7. Ibid.

8. Landers, *Encyclopedia,* p. 703.

9. U.S. Department of Health, Education and Welfare, *Report of the Secretary's Commission,* p. 9.

10. "Malpractice Awards," p. 79.

11. U.S. Department of Health, Education and Welfare, *Report of the Secretary's Commission,* p. 14.

12. *Wall Street Journal,* May 6, 1975.

13. Landers, *Encyclopedia,* p. 703.

14. American Medical Association, *Hospital Medical Staff Advocate* (Chicago, Ill.: AMA, 1979).

Chapter 21

Accreditation and Licensing

Key Terms

Joint Commission on Accreditation of Hospitals (JCAH) ∿ *Life safety code* ∿
Survey team ∿ *Licensure laws* ∿ *American Osteopathic Association (AOA)* ∿
American Hospital Association (AHA)

HISTORICAL REVIEW

How do patients and community residents know whether the hospital in their
community, or the hospital they are unfortunate enough to be a patient in, is a good
hospital? How does a patient know who has reviewed the systems, procedures,
physicians, nurses, and everything else in the hospital to make sure it is all working
properly? Fortunately, there is a group whose sole purpose is to review hospitals
and to tell hospitals, patients, and the community whether a hospital is satisfactory
or not. This process of review is called hospital accreditation, and the group that
does it is called the Joint Commission on Accreditation of Hospitals (JCAH). The
JCAH traces its roots to a program called the Hospital Standardization Program
that was established by the American College of Surgeons in 1918. The program
was established to enable surgeons to understand and appreciate the uniform
medical records format that would allow them to evaluate members who wished to
apply for fellowship status in the American College of Surgeons. From this
beginning, the group joined with four other groups—the American College of
Physicians, the American Medical Association, the American Hospital Association, and the American College of Surgeons—to form the JCAH. On January 1,
1952, the joint commission officially began its work of surveying hospitals and
granting accreditation. After its first year, it was clear that it had to have a more
dynamic nature, and its standards were amended slightly. Ever since that time the
joint commission has done a credible job of keeping up with new standards in this

country and constantly revising its approach to those standards. In the early years of the joint commission, up until 1961, the field studies were done by member organizations that were part of the JCAH. In 1961, the joint commission hired its own full-time field staff. In 1979, this staff surveyed over 2,000 hospitals.

In 1964 the joint commission began to charge a survey fee to the hospital in order to complete its field program. With the passage of Medicare legislation, Public Law 89-97, in 1965, the joint commission was given a big shot in the arm. It was written into the Medicare Act that hospitals participating under Medicare had to meet a certain level of quality of patient care as measured against a recognized norm. The JCAH was specifically referred to in the law and was asked to review hospitals for satisfactory participation. This was reaffirmed by the Social Security Administration in its standards of 1965.

All of this leads to three questions: What really is accreditation? What does accreditation mean to a hospital? How does a hospital become accredited?

THE ACCREDITATION PROCESS

How does a hospital become accredited? For a hospital to become accredited, it must first ask the JCAH, located in Chicago, to survey the hospital. The joint commission then sends the hospital a very large, involved, detailed questionnaire that cites the standards for a hospital. After the hospital has completed the questionnaire, a survey team is assigned, and a date is picked to visit the hospital.

The questionnaire, and thus the standards, are concerned with three major areas:

1. The physical plant and the environment in the hospital. This includes life-safety code problems, whether the hospital has adequate sprinkler systems, whether the corridors are large enough, whether there are proper safety exits, and the like.
2. The principles of organization and administration. Does the hospital have an effective bylaws structure? Does it have written policies and procedures? Does it require its departments to meet on a regular basis and to render written reports?
3. The services and quality of services the hospital renders to the patient. The JCAH reviews the nursing procedures, the dietary procedures, the pharmacy, the laboratory department, the x-ray department, and the emergency department services. It determines whether the services provided are truly adequate for the patient.

Recently, the joint commission has been spending a great deal of time and effort on quality assurance reviews in patient care areas. The surveyors review the patient's medical records to determine whether the doctors and nurses have given the care that was appropriate for that specific case.

WHAT DOES ACCREDITATION REALLY MEAN TO A HOSPITAL?

The hospital that has become accredited says to its community, its patients, and its employees that it wants to meet high standards and that it has taken the effort and time to have the joint commission come in to measure it against a set standard. Accreditation says to a hospital's employees and patients that the environment is of high quality and that the personnel are qualified to provide care. Lastly, accreditation says that the hospital is a responsible institution that takes its obligations for patient care seriously and has asked an independent, objective group to come in and review it.

HOW DOES A HOSPITAL BECOME ACCREDITED?

After the hospital completes the survey and the questionnaire, a JCAH survey team is scheduled to visit the hospital. The team consists of a physician, nurses, and sometimes a hospital administrator. If it is a large hospital, the survey team may consist of three members and usually take two days to complete the survey. If it is a small hospital, there may be two members (a physician and a nurse), and the survey may involve only a two-day visit.

The survey is quite complete and well organized. Each member of the survey team has a specific area to investigate and study. During the survey and inspection of the hospital, the surveyors write down in detail any deficiencies they observe in the hospital and then make certain recommendations. Before they leave the hospital, they give their list to the hospital administrator at a formal exit briefing. The survey team goes over with the administrator and key members of the administrator's staff exactly what they found that needs improvement and what they recommend. This is a very open, candid discussion on how the hospital can improve itself. The surveyor's list is then brought back to Chicago to JCAH headquarters where it is reviewed in detail. Finally, a decision is made, based upon the survey, whether the hospital should be accredited and whether the accreditation should be for one year or two years. Approximately 60 percent of the hospitals in this country receive a two-year accreditation, the balance receive a one-year accreditation; 3 to 5 percent are not certified at all.

After a hospital has been accredited by the JCAH, it receives a certificate of accreditation indicating this achievement. If it receives a two-year accreditation, it must in the interim year before the next JCAH visit complete a detailed questionnaire identifying what it has done about the deficiencies noted in the original questionnaire. The interim questionnaire is sent to the joint commission in Chicago where it is evaluated.

In summary, the JCAH fills a major void in the evaluation of hospitals in this country. It is a unique organization in a world in which the government and bureaucracy legislate everything. The JCAH has been responsive to the hospitals and to the federal government through Medicare; it provides a silent service to the patient and community; it maintains high professional standards; it acts as an advisory group to hospitals and has been influential in urging hospitals to improve their life safety measures, their quality assurance programs, and their organizations.

The JCAH has been a success. It is unique in the health care arena and in the hospital setting because it is a voluntary operation whose goal is to make sure that the patients going into the hospital are served with the quality and dignity they deserve.

LICENSURE

Though the JCAH review and inspection are the primary controls over the hospitals in a licensing sense—particularly since the federal government under Titles XVIII and XIX of the Medicare legislation, Public Law 89-97, has endorsed the joint commission's survey in order to certify payment for hospitals under the Medicare legislation—there are other forms of control working in the hospital system.

Since the enactment of the Hospital Construction (Hill-Burton) Act in 1946, many states have instituted state licensing laws and regulations for hospitals. A federal government report indicates that there are almost 500 state agencies in the United States that have licensing, approval, certification, and supervisory regulations for inpatient hospitals and related health care facilities.[1] There were some 53 regulatory agencies with authority over short-stay hospitals and another 52 regulatory agencies with authority over psychiatric hospitals.

Licensing is the most common form of regulation by the states. Generally a license to operate a hospital is issued by a state agency, perhaps the welfare department or the health department in the state. Generally, the licensing bureau or agency retains records of a hospital's bed capacity and the capacities of its other facilities. The health and welfare departments of the states account for three-quarters of the state agencies that have regulatory powers over hospitals. A state's licensure laws and regulations usually culminate in a licensure inspection that is similar to the inspection conducted by the JCAH. Therein lies one of the overlaps in the regulatory system. Frequently, state inspectors and joint commission inspectors inspect the same things, sometimes within the same month or within the same short period of time. Thus the cry from hospital administrators that they are being "inspected to death."

CERTIFICATION

Another form of control used for hospitals beyond licensure is the process of certification. Hospitals have had to deal with the issue of certification since the 1965 Social Security Amendments that sponsored Title XVIII and Title XIX. At that time, the government established a way for hospitals to participate in the federal insurance programs but indicated that they had to meet certain general compliance conditions in order to do so, for example, establish an around-the-clock nursing staff, certain medical supervision, and the proper use of clinical records. Essentially, certification has become associated with the joint commission's annual or biannual surveys. It should be noted that the American Osteopathic Association (AOA) certifies osteopathic hospitals through inspection reports under the Medicare program.

REGISTRATION

Registration is a weak form of control in the system. Indeed, it may not even be regarded by hospital authorities as a control. However, there is a system of registration that identifies hospitals and other health care institutions so that the third parties, consumers, and federal agencies can review the rosters of such institutions. The most common registration in the hospital system is conducted by the American Hospital Association (AHA). The AHA maintains an extensive system of data collection in the form of hospital profiles. It is also involved in registering hospitals in planning areas; for example, new construction, proposed mergers, or the sharing of services are all reviewed by the AHA. The AHA publishes an annual hospital statistics report that includes data from much of its registration activities.

NOTE

1. U.S. Department of Health, Education and Welfare, "Part II, Inpatient Health Facilities," *Health Resources Statistics 1972-73*, DHEW, 1973, publication no. 73-1509, p. 347.

Part IX

Continuing To Grow

Chapter 22

Hospital Marketing

Key Terms

Marketing philosophy ∼ Physician recruiting ∼ Exchange relationships ∼ Marketing audit ∼ Market segments ∼ Concept of positioning ∼ The four Ps ∼ The public relations department ∼ Internal publications ∼ Fund raising ∼ Hospital advertising

INTRODUCTION

The idea of a hospital involved in marketing may seem at first glance to be crass and inappropriate. In the past, marketing has been associated with businesses and retail activities, certainly not with hospital service. It could in fact be argued that hospital care is something everybody needs and therefore should not have to be marketed or sold at all. On the other hand, the case could be made that hospital care has already been oversold to America and that what is truly needed is more health maintenance or more attention to personal habits, life styles, and environmental factors.

Hospitals, like the rest of the health care field, have traditionally avoided marketing and marketing efforts. They have looked askance at advertising and competitive pricing, though they have been willing to make some attempts in improving their public and community relations. Yet, by avoiding direct association with the marketing process, a hospital may well fall into the trap of being unresponsive to its market—its patients and potential patients.

Though marketing is becoming a "buzz" word in the hospital area, the record shows that since 1975 no more than 10 percent of the nation's 7,000 hospitals have established formal marketing programs or hired marketing directors.[1] Hospitals have tended to shy away from the marketing approach in their planning and development efforts. The prevailing philosophy has been to let people make their selection of services through their own physicians. In short, the hospital does not need to decide in advance how to attract patients. This is hardly a marketing philosophy.

Marketing suggests that hospitals should try to determine its public needs and that it should attempt to meet these needs by developing appropriate programs. A close look at the situation indicates that in that sense some hospitals really do market in some areas, though they may not call it that. Perhaps the best example is in the area of physician recruiting. Many hospitals avidly recruit physicians to join their medical staffs. The hospital is willing to give to the recruited physicians certain benefits, for example, the right to practice in the hospital or medical office building, special parking spaces, and the like.

Thus, in the critical matter of physician recruiting and maintaining an active, adequate, loyal hospital medical staff, a classic marketing function is at work. In the physician recruiting process, there is a voluntary exchange of values between two parties, the hospital and the physicians. The hospital needs what the physician has, namely, the licensed ability to admit and to manage the care of the patient. From the other side, the physician needs what the hospital has, namely, admitting privileges, up-to-date equipment, and a well-trained ancillary and support staff. In the recruiting process, both parties have exchanged things; in so doing, they have also become a part of the marketing process.

Hospitals must study this marketing matter very closely. The U.S. government estimates that there are 130,000 excess beds in the country that cost Americans 2 billion dollars a year. It has been predicted that within the next five years between 1,000 and 1,500 hospitals will close in this country.[2] These statistics suggest that hospital managers should become sensitive to what marketing and the marketing process can do to help hospitals.

WHAT IS MARKETING?

To paraphrase William J. Stanton, professor of marketing at the University of Colorado, marketing is a total system of interacting management activities that are designed to plan, price, promote, and distribute need- and want-satisfying services to a hospital's present and potential patients.[3] According to another definition, "managing or planning simple exchange relationships" is the essence of marketing.[4] In this exchange definition of marketing, the purchase behavior can be viewed as a simple exchange of resources, that is, a certain individual gives another individual something in order to receive in exchange a privilege, a good, or a service. Note how this definition relates closely to the physician recruiting example used earlier.

MARKETING CONCEPTS

Hospitals must become familiar with certain key concepts in the marketing process if they are to be successful in their marketing efforts. Perhaps the best place to begin is with the marketing audit. A marketing audit is simply a systematic, objective, critical way of appraising how the hospital is relating to its markets at any given point in time. The purpose of the marketing audit is to establish a basis on which to decide what kind of marketing program can be developed. There are three simple steps in the marketing audit:

1. The hospital must identify the kinds of information it wishes to gather in order to evaluate its market or patient relations.
2. It must set about collecting this data and information.
3. It then must evaluate the data and information it has collected.

Perhaps the standard marketing audit employed by hospitals is the physician audit. After a marketing audit has been completed, it may become clear to the hospital that it has more than one kind of audience or public.

The various audiences that the hospital works with are called segments or market segments. A market segment is a distinct group of patients or potential patients that can be separated from another group. For example, it is very common to divide patients by type of insurance—Medicare, Medicaid, or Blue Cross. It is also common to divide patients by age. Frequently, patients are divided by income level or by geographic location. The different ways of categorizing the hospital's patients identify particular market segments.

After completing an audit and identifying a hospital's different segments, it is important for the hospital to realize that it has an image among the patients and also among its competing hospitals. Where the hospital fits into this image spectrum is called the hospital's position. The concept of positioning is important to understand when trying to determine what programs the hospital should invest in and sponsor. To use an illustration from the business arena, the Avis position was not clear until the company finally adopted the slogan that they were number two. This move had great success precisely because Avis did not position itself directly opposite its number one competitor but in fact differentiated itself from its competition. Put into hospital language, if a neighboring hospital has a superior cardiology unit, perhaps the first hospital should do something in outpatient pediatrics. It would thereby position itself as different from a competitor that is successful and strong.

With this concept of a marketing audit, segment, and position in mind, the marketing program can proceed with the classic four Ps of marketing. The objective is to put the right *product* in the hospital's case service into the right *place* (proper location) at the right *price* with the proper *promotion*.

With regard to the right product, it should be remembered that hospitals do not really sell services; rather they sell the benefits of satisfaction the patients get from receiving services. This is the hospital's product. Ideally, a hospital should conduct inventories or marketing audits frequently to determine what its product and benefits should be. Hospitals should regularly analyze their service programs.

With regard to the marketing place, the best example in the hospital field can be seen in satellite outpatient clinics or in medical office buildings that are placed near a hospital. Such hospitals have placed their services in the right location. They are convenient to the market.

With respect to price, because of the way the federal government reimburses the hospital for care, prices have become less important to the hospital industry than to retail businesses. There is still, however, a psychology of price. For example, the market is somewhat sensitive to price for an hour in the operating room, for a four-days' stay in the nursery, or for a standard charge for a CBC or urinalysis. Thus price still must be considered in the total marketing program.

The last "P," promotion, refers to the classic public relations activities that hospitals have undertaken. It also refers to advertising and to other innovative ways of promoting products (for example, premiums and incentives that could be offered to certain people). Hospitals need administrators, trustees, and public relations staff members who are sensitive to promotional issues in health services.

It is important for hospitals to understand in detail the strategies and tactics of the marketing process. If they want to attract new physicians, to develop effective programs, to retain qualified personnel, and to stay up-to-date in their delivery services, marketing can be a great asset.

ELEMENTS OF MARKETING

There are two elements of marketing that hospitals are getting involved in more and more. One is a traditional element; the other is something for the future. The traditional element is hospital public relations. The future element is in advertising.

Public Relations

Public relations has been defined by Webster as "the art or science of developing reciprocal understanding and goodwill between a person, firm, or institution and the public. . . ."[5] Another definition of public relations is "the activities of an organization in building and maintaining sound relations with specific publics such as customer, employer, etc., and with the public at large so as to adapt to its environment and interpret itself to society."[6]

For many years, hospitals have understood the need to develop and retain positive relationships with their patients, their potential donors, and their community at large. This is in contrast to the newer concept of advertising that hospitals are not yet familiar with and are just starting to explore. Unfortunately for hospitals, public relations is a great deal more difficult to target to specific market segments than is advertising. However, public relations can improve a hospital's image, generate the public's interest, and aid in fund-raising efforts.

Most hospitals are likely to have some sort of formal or informal public relations program. Some may even have a full-time public relations staff. The main objective of this staff is to arrange for the hospital to receive favorable publicity in the community. The staff can do different things to accomplish this. They might invite a local newspaper editor to join their board, thereby improving the chances of favorable publicity. Or they could develop strong contacts with a local television and radio station.

The Need for Public Relations

Most large hospitals have formal public relations activities or a public relations department. The public relations department is a staff or advisory department. Generally, there is a public relations director in charge of the department. The PR Department works closely with all other departments in the hospital, but the public relations function is clearly the responsibility of the hospital management. The technical aspects of public relations, such as developing brochures or writing press releases, is usually left to a technical expert. A public relations program need not necessarily be costly or elaborate, but it must be well thought out and systematically developed with management input if it is to be effective and get the message across in a proper manner.

A community hospital has two constituents. The first is an internal public—the hospital's board of trustees, its employees, its medical staff members, its volunteers, and "friends" of the hospital. This internal public is relatively easy to target and penetrate with the hospital's positive public image. This is usually accomplished through a series of traditional publications.

The most difficult segment to reach is the hospital's external public. This consists of potential patients of the hospital, the hospital's community, and the potential fund-raising contributors of the hospital. This public is not as clearly defined and is a much more difficult challenge for public relations directors and hospital management.

Publications

Most hospitals are involved in publishing public relations material and literature for their internal group. Hospitals commonly publish booklets containing patient or employee information. Frequently, they publish their own internal newspapers, institutional brochures, or even annual reports for the internal group. Most of these publications are initiated by the hospital administrator and management team. The hospital's patient audience has the greatest need for this type of published material and information, but, unfortunately for the hospital, the hospital has only a brief period in which to get its message across to its patients.

Traditional internal publications may include the following:

- A patient's information booklet. This booklet contains information that familiarizes the patient with the hospital's environment, gives the do's and don't's of being a patient, and focuses on visitor information.

- An employee information handbook. This gives the employee the rules of employment, lists the employee's rights and obligations, and frequently outlines in some detail the fringe benefits available as an employee.

- A hospital newsletter. Typically this is done by a local printer and is not generally of the quality of the mass media that most of us are familiar with. The newsletter may be published infrequently, perhaps once a month or once a quarter. The reporting staff is usually made up of amateur writers and reporters from within the hospital. However, it is a source of information, and, if done properly, employee groups enjoy reading it.

- An institutional brochure. This is available to internal groups, the board of trustees, and volunteers. It usually presents the history of the hospital, the philosophy of the institution, and other interesting facets of the hospital's operation.

- The annual report. When a hospital publishes a formal annual report, it is usually done with quality printing and a high degree of expertise in its layout. The report is used for internal purposes of the medical staff, board of trustees, and employees and is frequently sent to other hospitals and to some elements of the external public. Annual reports summarize the operational highlights of the year and usually list the key management team and medical staff.

Perhaps the most common relationship with the hospital's outside public is through the mass media or press relations. The mass media provide a means of getting the hospital's message to the community. The hospital has specific objectives it wants to accomplish—mainly to keep its outside public informed, to improve or build a positive image for the hospital in the community, and to attempt to gain some influence on what the mass media report in the health care arena. Press releases are commonly used by the public relations department to keep in touch with the mass media.

When a hospital embarks upon a capital fund-raising campaign or annual fund-raising effort, it must solicit its public, usually in written form. Though hospitals may not consider this a function of public relations, it clearly is, since many letters of solicitation are sent out. Often, costly folders or brochures are developed and sent out, usually through direct mail to gain a specific reaction, namely, to raise funds from the hospital's external public.

Hospital Advertising

Unlike the traditional public relations role of a hospital, advertising is a relatively new concept in the health care area. Advertising has been defined in different ways by different people. The American Marketing Association has described it as "mass, paid communications whose purpose is to impart information, develop attitudes, and induce favorable action for the advertiser."[7] Hospitals have been relatively slow in adapting the advertising process to their field. Typically, they have been satisfied with public relations efforts or unpaid statements that are printed in newspapers or magazines or given over radio and television. However, some approaches, such as the distribution of annual reports to external groups, border on advertising in some ways, since they are skillfully done and forwarded to specific target markets. Unfortunately, advertising still arouses considerable controversy in the hospital field. It conjures up unethical or even illegal practices. Much of this is mythical. In fact, advertising has a major role to play in the entire marketing process, in both not-for-profit and profitmaking activities in this country. Hospitals are finding that they can have advertising tailored to their professional needs and can select very specific markets for mailings. For example, they can target their advertising efforts on physicians who may be interested in using the hospital. Frequently, hospitals think about advertising as a way to improve activity in a lesser-used service of the hospital. For example, prospective obstetrical patients may be attracted by a family-centered maternity room that has been advertised in the mass media.

Functions

In general, hospital advertising (1) informs the public, (2) persuades the public, and (3) reminds the public. Mass production has created an economy of abundance. In this context, hospitals are competitive institutions. The federal government reports that there are too many hospital beds in this country. In this situation it is logical to conclude that hospitals will turn to what our for-profit retailing cousins have learned, namely, that people can be persuaded to use one service over another. People can select those services that they want to receive. The hospital can make its product or service known and tell about its benefits and features. Then it can use advertising to remind the publics who have used that service to continue to use the service. It can remind them of the reasons they were satisfied with the hospital and what brought them there in the first place. These functions of advertising are just now being applied by hospitals. Initially hospitals may develop their advertising around public information or public educational vehicles. In years to come, these efforts will provide a fertile and growing field for hospital advertising.

What are some of the reasons for hospitals to advertise? First of all, the hospital's patients may need information on how to prevent disease and illness, for example, guidance on good nutrition or on how a woman can administer breast examinations herself. A second reason is that hospital patients need to understand the health care system and how preventive medicine and preventive programs interact with health care professionals, for example, where cancer screening may be available and why and where children can receive immunizations. Hospitals are becoming more involved in such programs. A third reason is that hospital patients need to be informed on how to use properly all of the elements in the health care system. Hospital advertising can deliver this type of information and in so doing improve the image not only of the hospital from which the advertising is sent but the entire hospital industry's image as well. Hospitals are likely to be interested in advertising along these lines, since such efforts are very closely related to their mission of health education.

Outside Agencies' Positions on Advertising

Hospitals may differ in the quality of service they provide or in the uniqueness of the services they offer. According to the American Hospital Association, hospital advertising is legitimate when it includes facts related to hospital services and to space facilities. The American Hospital Association's position is that it is ethical for a hospital to make its public aware of any unused services. However, the association draws the line at comparative advertising. Yet, comparative advertising will likely become more and more common, and the guidelines of the American Hospital Association may have to be altered or bent to accommodate the change.

It is important to note that the federal government, through Medicare legislation, has stated its position on advertising by a provider: advertising ". . . is an allowable cost if it is a necessary part of the provider's operation and therefore appropriate and helpful in furnishing covered services to many care beneficiaries."[8] Note that the government's position on advertising is very close to that of the American Hospital Association's guidelines. However, the Medicare rules specify that costs incurred by a hospital to increase its patient service utilization are *not* allowable for Medicare reimbursement. For example, Medicare will not allow costs that compensate institutions, hospitals, or physicians for the admission of patients to the hospital, and it will not underwrite costs to influence these parties to refer patients to a given hospital.

An interesting aspect of advertising that has come to the attention of the federal government is that of yellow-page directory advertising. Depending on the specific nature of such advertising, the federal government under Medicare may or may not allow it. For example, the basic entry in simple alphabetical listings is allowable. However, if the advertisement is an elaborate, skillfully laid out piece with bold headings and pictures, most likely the cost will not be reimbursed.

The Future of Hospital Advertising

More hospital administrators are seeking help from advertising to meet their marketing problems. Much of this advertising will be geared to consumers as it has been in the past. However, it may be directed at physicians and other hospitals and institutions as well. There may, indeed, be a tendency in the future to overestimate how effective advertising can be for a hospital. Thus, administrators will have to evaluate carefully the cost benefits of advertising. In conclusion, lucrative advertising is just beginning to enter the area of hospital marketing. In the future, hospitals and hospital management will increasingly use advertising by adapting and tailoring it to the unique needs of the hospital field.

NOTES

1. Thomas Livingston, ed., *Executive Memo,* Saga Dietary Company, September 1979, p. 1.
2. Ibid.
3. William Stanton, *Fundamentals of Marketing* (New York, N.Y.: McGraw-Hill Book Company, 1975), p. 5.
4. Tim Garton, "Marketing Health Care: Its Untapped Potential," *Hospital Progress,* February 1973, p. 46.
5. *Webster's New Collegiate Dictionary,* 7th ed., s.v. "public relations."
6. "Marketing Insights," April 7, 1969.
7. Harvey R. Cook, *Selecting Advertising Media, A Guide for Small Business* (Washington, D.C.: U.S. Government Printing Office, 1969), p. 1.
8. U.S. Department of Health, Education and Welfare, May 1979, "Part A Intermediary Letter No. 79-22," p. 1.

Long-Range Planning

Key Terms

Section 1122 review process ~ *Regional Comprehensive Health Planning Agencies (RCHPA)* ~ *Public Law 93-641, Health Systems Agencies (1975)* ~ *Certificate of need* ~ *Demographic profile* ~ *Health status indicators* ~ *Satterfield Amendment*

INTRODUCTION

The concept of planning is basic to the management of the hospital. Planning makes management sense, and common sense as well, particularly now when third parties and regulatory agencies are pushing the hospital into more sophisticated and formal planning. Hospitals are in the midst of a rapidly changing environment. Hospital managers look around and see the demands of the population are changing. The need for physicians is increasing. The matter of solvency and appropriate reimbursement mandates budgetary planning. Add to this the fact that hospitals are becoming more and more competitive. In this situation, the hospital's survival is truly contingent upon its ability to make the right informed strategic decisions for its future course of action.

Over the last ten years, hospital planning has changed its focus entirely. Through the 1960s, planning was generally synonymous with developing new facilities in a rapidly expanding health care market. Today, partly because of the oversupply of beds in many areas and the tightening of government regulations, planning may mean a great deal more than expansion and growth. Today, planning is used to ensure that a hospital's services are necessary and appropriate and that those services will thrive in the future. Recently it has become common for hospitals to develop associations, shared services, or linkages with other health providers as part of their planning process.

Hospitals are looking seriously at horizontal growth in the industry. For example, they are exploring home care, primary care, long-term care, and other forms of subacute care that relate directly to the hospital. Many hospitals are joining together in not-for-profit multisystems of one type or another. This is surprising, in view of the fact that only ten years ago almost all nonprofit hospitals were freestanding. It has been estimated that one-third of the nation's 6,500 community general hospitals are now in some sort of shared system.

THE NEED FOR PLANNING AGENCIES

Basic economics teaches us that as the price of a certain service or good is reduced and approaches zero, the demand for that service or good begins to reach infinity. Therein lies the gist of the economic fallacy in the Medicare and Medicaid programs of 1966: Congress allowed reimbursement on "reasonable cost" rather than on competitive market cost. The patients on Medicare and Medicaid and other third party payers do not really believe they are paying directly for their services. By taking the element of direct cost away from the consumer, the classic economics of supply and demand in hospitals has become confused.

After the first year of the Medicare and Medicaid programs, in 1967, their expenditures totaled 5 billion dollars; ten years later, in 1977, they exceeded 33 billion dollars. It was at that point that Congress reconsidered its generosity and initiated legislation to reduce hospital costs in an attempt to contain the costs of the programs. Congress had a feeling that hospitals and other providers, by adding layers of facilities and personnel onto the Medicare and Medicaid programs, were attempting too much in the health care system. There was a feeling that what was needed to contain the rising costs was health planning legislation. Thus, in 1971, Congress passed the Social Security Act with Section 1122 (review process) of Public Law 92-603. This law established Regional Comprehensive Health Planning Agencies (RCHPA). These regulations became effective in 1972. After a few years of experience with the RCHPA program, however, Congress saw that hospitals were still being constructed at a vigorous pace. Additional legislation, in the form of Public Law 93-641, followed in 1975. This law dissolved the Regional Comprehensive Health Planning Agencies created in 1971 and replaced them with Health Systems Agencies (HSAs). Other elements in the earlier law were tightened up, and a certificate of need (CON) for new equipment and facilities over $100,000 became mandatory.

EARLY PLANNING EFFORTS

One of the earliest planning efforts at the community level was the Hospital Council of Greater New York, which was established in 1938 to meet the needs for community agencies to plan and to coordinate hospital facilities and services in

New York City. In 1948, a planning agency was initiated in Philadelphia, but it was discontinued in 1952. The record shows that in 1954 at least ten hospital councils, located mostly in large urban cities, had made some progress on capital planning in their respective regions. After 1955, more and more agencies were specifically structured to aid in community planning, and definite planning programs were set up for metropolitan hospital areas. For example, in 1957, the Detroit Area Hospital Council and the Kansas City Area Hospital Council Association established planning programs.

The issue of planning attempts during the 1950s was accurately summarized by Leroy E. Burney, Surgeon General of the United States Public Health Service, when he said: "Of one thing I am reasonably certain, no one organization or type of institution in this country today has the breadth of experience or has shown the initiative required for developing the whole range of health facilities and services the American people should have."[1] Because the hospitals have not been effective in their planning, at least from the government's standpoint, the hospital system is today saddled with layer upon layer of regulations concerning cost containment and hospital and health services planning.

THE HOSPITAL'S LONG-RANGE PLAN

Hospitals are now required by federal laws and a variety of state laws to develop institutional long-range planning. There is a federal requirement that hospitals who receive Medicare and Medicaid funds must plan as required in the Social Security Amendments of 1972, Public Law 92-603. In this legislation, under Section 234 of the Act, proper hospital planning requires an annual operating budget, capital expenditures to be identified and detailed for at least three years, and anticipated sources of financing and anticipated expenditures in excess of $100,000. A review and updating of these plans must be made at least annually. The governing body under a planning committee, including the administration and medical staff, must oversee the preparation of these plans.

Although the government essentially forces the hospital to do strategic planning, it is actually to the advantage of a hospital to do sound, practical planning for the future—particularly now when there are so many forces (competitors to the hospital and other health agencies) impacting on a hospital's environment that must be considered by the board of trustees and hospital management. The changing patterns of medical practice include the shift from acute inpatients to ambulatory medicine, the mushrooming of biomedical technology with its impact on the hospital's operation and future, and shifts in demography and community needs. These changing patterns are especially important in urban areas where age and racial mix and mobility are constant factors in hospital planning. Finally, changing economic conditions—particularly in the availability of money to carry out the hospital's plans—and increased legislation and regulations will impact the hospital. All of these factors must be placed into the planning mix in order to come up with a menu that will serve the hospital in the future.

WHO SHOULD DO THE HOSPITAL'S PLANNING?

The hospital should have a long-range planning committee. It is a vehicle for sound management as well as being stipulated in Public Law 92-603. It was Section 1122 of this legislation that denied federal reimbursement under the Medicare and Medicaid programs for any unapproved expenditures. This committee should have representatives from the board of trustees, the hospital administration, and the medical staff. However, the best plans will also require input from community members so that the community's needs and the tone of the community can be identified. The name of the committee may vary; it may be called the long-range planning committee, the planning committee, or some other name. The committee's functions must include those outlined in Public Law 92-603. Typically the size of the committee will range from 8 to 12 members—a manageable size, yet large enough for a variety of viewpoints and inputs. Members of the board of trustees who are members of the committee should reflect the hospital's intent and commitment to long-range planning. In addition, if they themselves are not community members, they should make sure that the community is represented in the long-range planning process. The board must approve the final long-range plan.

The administrator or CEO has the job of guiding the committee through the long-range planning process. As the person who is primarily responsible for carrying out the board's decisions, the administrator or CEO participates actively in the planning deliberations. Usually, the administrator determines the planning process that will be followed and suggests various options available to the board in making long-range planning decisions.

The medical staff's role is also critical. The medical staff must identify changes in the health care needs of the community and suggest new options on how the hospital might meet these changing medical needs. Medical staff members are spokespersons for the advancing medical technology and can advise the board's planning committee on how this technology will impact the hospital's plan. Another byproduct of having the medical staff participate in the committee is that staff members can become acquainted with the problems facing the hospital management in planning for the future, usually in an environment of limited resources.

CONTENTS OF A LONG-RANGE PLAN

Hospitals will vary in how they write their plans and in what will be included. However, elements that should be included in any long-range plan are:

- a demographic profile of the hospital's community

- health status indicators of the area

- the hospital's relationships to other health care services and providers

- specific hospital data—namely, patient origins, professional staff, utilization patterns, and financial data

- forecasts of all important statistical and related data

- an examination of the external forces that may affect the hospital in the future

- the admission statement of the hospital

- specific goals and quantifiable objectives for the future

- selected courses and alternative courses of action

- the selected course of action

- strategies for implementing the plan

- specifics of certificate-of-need forecasts, including not only major building programs but major equipment that might be needed in the hospital.

BENEFITS FROM PLANNING

Clearly, proper long-range planning will improve the hospital's overall ability to deal with the future. Specifically, it will show benefits in these areas:

- It will establish a systematic basis for relating to the allocation of specific and frequently limited resources in the hospital's future.

- It will ensure that the hospital continues to look at its admission statement and its resources to carry out its mission.

- It will continue to test the viability of the hospital by integrating budgets with long-range strategic plans.

- It will give management more control because it will have a better idea of where it is going; this will also guide management's day-to-day operations.

- It will give the hospital a standard for management against which performance can then be evaluated and measured.

GOVERNMENT CONTROL

In 1979, Congress passed Public Law 96-79, the Health Planning and Resource Development Amendments. This was the first significant health planning legislation since Public Law 93-641 was passed in 1974. This new legislation will affect all aspects of health planning, including certificates of need, health system plans, and health systems agency governing bodies. The legislation frees hospitals from being held captive by a Health Systems Agency (HSA) during the hospital's planning processes. Under the Satterfield Amendment to the legislation, most of the flagrant abuses of the planning process have been cut away, for example, the alleged holding of certain hospitals hostage by some health systems agencies in the review process in order to extract changes in their institutional complement of beds or plans that were unrelated to their reason for going to the agency for planning approval. This legislation essentially culminated a ten-year effort on the government's part to save money in the health planning process.

A recent survey by the American Health Planning Association, a private group formed in 1971 to encourage planning activities, shows that "one-and-a-half billion dollars a year in hospital and nursing home capital expenditures is being denied or diverted by the Health Planning Agency."[2] The report showed that a proposed 5,717 short-term hospital beds were disapproved by the agencies over a two-year period. Based on this report and other less well documented evidence, the health planning agencies and the government's interest in planning clearly are having an impact on hospital costs. We can conclude that the impact in the future will be even greater. A brief chronology of government involvement in health planning is provided in Exhibit 23-1.

BUILDING A NEW HOSPITAL

Frequently the stimulation for and the culmination of a hospital planning effort is the construction of a major addition, a new wing, or a completely new hospital. To build a new hospital successfully, the administration, the board of trustees, and those consultants they select to assist them must follow a specifically outlined course through the construction program. Successful hospital projects generally include the following phases: (1) planning, (2) programming, (3) design, (4) construction, and (5) financing. Although the financing phase is listed last, this phase must be finalized before construction actually begins. The American Hospital Association has published a booklet *Building a Hospital, A Primer for Administrators,* by John Rea et al. This is an easy-to-read, comprehensive work that outlines many of the issues a hospital board of trustees and administrator should understand before beginning a major construction program. With the planning phase out of the way, the other tasks in the building project can then be launched.

Exhibit 23-1 Chronology of Major Federal Health Planning Legislation

---

1946—*The Hospital Survey and Construction Act (Hill-Burton)* provided, among other things, for the creation of a state hospital planning council to assess the need for new hospital construction and to develop a plan indicating priorities to meet these needs.

1961—*The Community Health Services and Facilities Act,* among other things, provided grants for voluntary health facility planning agencies at the local level.

1964—*The Hospital and Medical Facilities Amendments (Hill-Harris Act, P.L. 88-443)* provided funds for modernization or replacement of health care facilities, as well as additional funds for facility planning purposes. In addition, the law provided matching funds for the purpose of establishing health facility planning agencies in areas where there had been none before.

1966—*The Comprehensive Health Planning and Public Health Service Amendments (P.L. 89-749)* provided health revenue sharing funds for state governments, plus grants for comprehensive health planning at the state and local level.

1972—*The Social Security Amendments of 1972 (P.L. 92-603)* added, among other things, Sections 234 and 1122 to the Social Security Act. Section 234 requires institutional planning by hospitals, extended care facilities, and home health agencies as a condition for participating in Medicare. Section 1122 provides, in participating states, that health care facilities and HMOs will not be reimbursed by Medicare (Title XVIII), Medicaid (Title XIX), or the Maternal and Child Health Programs (Title V) for depreciation, interest, and return on equity capital relating to capital expenditures that are determined by designated state agencies to be unnecessary

Exhibit 23-1 continued

1975—*The National Health Planning and Resources Development
Act of 1974 (P.L. 93-641)* amends the Public Health Service
Act by adding Titles XV and XVI. Title XV revises existing
health planning programs at the state and area-wide level and
encourages the Secretary of HEW to work on the development
of national health policy. Title XVI revises the Hill-Burton program for the construction and modernization of health care
facilities by linking the award for grants and loans to the mechanisms created in Title XV.

1979—*Health Planning and Resources Development Amendments
of 1979 (P.L. 96-79).* This was an extensive package of
amendments to P.L. 93-641. The new legislation affects all
aspects of health planning, including certificate of need, health
systems plans, and HSA governing bodies. The legislation
also includes a section referred to as the Satterfield Amendment, which was proposed to cure an abuse in the earlier
planning process. The Satterfield Amendment prohibits the
HSAs from using the review process to have hospitals take
actions that are unrelated to the subject of the hospital's application.

NOTES

1. Joseph K. Owen, *Modern Concepts of Hospital Administration* (Philadelphia, Pa.: W.B. Saunders Co., 1962), p. 51.
2. William Boyles, ''Health Planning Agencies Save $1.5 Billion a Year: Study,'' *Health Care Week,* January 1, 1979, p. 1.

The Elements of a Health Care System

Chapter 24

The Medical Care System

Key Terms

A medical system ᵜ Solo practitioner ᵜ "Medicaid mills" ᵜ Medically indigent ᵜ Maldistribution of physicians ᵜ Teaching hospitals ᵜ Ambulance services ᵜ Community hospitals ᵜ Skilled nursing facilities (SNFs) ᵜ Intermediate care facilities (ICFs) ᵜ Consumers

INTRODUCTION

Webster defines a system as a "set or arrangement of things so related or connected as to form a unity or organic whole; a set of principles, etc., arranged in a regular orderly form as to show a logical plan linking the various parts."[1] More specifically, a health or medical system is a set of mechanisms through which human resources, facilities, and medical technology are organized by means of administrative structures. The system offers integrated services in sufficient quantity and quality to meet the community's demand at a cost compatible with the community's financial resources.

The American medical system offers three classes of care: middle-class care given to approximately 185 million Americans; second-class care, available to approximately 21 million poor people; and the narrow and limited "princely" care given to the elite and super-wealthy. Because our society has much more knowledge than know-how, there has been prodigious progress in medical science but a failure to make it accessible in equal proportions to all segments of our society.

The type of medical care a person receives depends upon where the person lives and how much money the person has. Better care is given to those living near university medical centers or the sophisticated urban teaching hospitals. A fact of American life is that medicine has been and still remains a middle class institution.

235

Of course, physicians practice on the poor, but they are really concentrated on taking care of the middle class.

In this chapter we will describe, but not defend, the medical care system (or the sickness system) that exists in this country today. The different components or elements of the system will be examined. There are four medical institutional elements that are related; and there is one additional element, the community.

THE SYSTEM'S GOALS

Before examining each of the components in detail, it is appropriate to keep in mind the general goals of our national health care system. These goals are presently being met in varying degrees, depending on the geographic locale and the economic status of the individual. Some of the gaps in the medical care system are seen when the goals are weighed against what is actually happening in the medical world. In short, the traditional American medical system has aimed at the following goals:

- The system should be available to all the people.

- The system should be both psychologically and socially acceptable to all those using it.

- The system should have quality.

- The system should be comprehensive and stress maximum economy.

With these goals in mind, let us examine the various components of the medical care system.

OUTREACH ELEMENT

The first component of the medical care system is the outreach element. In essence, the traditional system attempts to meet the patient's primary medical care needs through outreach programs. These programs are generally decentralized. They are scattered activities. Outpatient activities include health care centers, group practices, ambulatory care arrangements, and outpatient activities of health maintenance organizations (HMOs), among other activities.

Traditionally, most patients in America have received care through their primary care physician (or the solo practitioner). This is the most common example of the system's outreach component. Private or solo practitioners provide the bulk of the American outreach activity. At the same time, the urban poor use city health clinics, public health nurses, or visiting nurses associations. The outreach element also includes groups like school nurses, sophisticated group practices that are free-standing from hospitals, the myriad of storefront clinics that are found in urban centers, and the multispecialty offices in the inner city called "Medicaid mills" that proliferate in some of our urban areas. Other social agencies have from time to time been involved in the outreach component. Churches often are involved in screening activities and in providing centers for referral through physicians or hospitals. This outreach phase is the beginning of the referral sequence for many patients in our present medical care system.

In the outreach component we are able to distinguish two classes of care. As we have noted, one type of care is offered to the 185 million middle-class consumers; the other is given to the 21 million poor among us. These two groups take different routes in the outreach element. The middle class historically has been served by the private practitioner and the primary care physician. Presently, there are 194 physicians per 100,000 population in America, but only 65 primary care physicians per 100,000 population.[2]

The record shows that there is a maldistribution of physicians; urban areas and ghettos as well as our depressed rural areas have a paucity of physicians. Rarely do you find members of the middle class using city health clinics, neighborhood health centers, or mental health program clinics. It is much more common for the medically indigent to use these sites. The real and significant difference between the two populations is how the middle class and the poor class are referred into the rest of the medical institutions in the system. Clearly, the two groups are not referred with the same social and psychological acceptance. Thus, the outreach component of our traditional system is in trouble. Indeed, an increasing problem is that the middle class is also having difficulty being referred into the other sectors of the medical care system. Even middle class patients now have difficulty finding primary care practitioners in their quiet suburban areas. Simply put, middle-class consumers cannot guide themselves through the medical care system. The patients want physicians to take care of the whole person, not just the orthopedic, urologic, or psychiatric problem. This new problem for the middle class is the same one that our poor have experienced for years. Now that the entire system, and especially the outreach component, is coming under attack, perhaps there will be a change.

OUTPATIENT ELEMENT

The second component of our health care system is the outpatient component. This is the part of the system that embodies the traditional hospital clinics. Historically, the clinics located in large urban areas were created for teaching purposes or to service the poor. The outpatient element also embraces the mushrooming emergency departments across the nation. It also includes the ambulance squads: the municipal police and firemen and the suburban community ambulance services. In addition, hospital-based group practices are included in this element.

In analyzing the outpatient component we have to recognize that there are differences between clinics. Those that are associated with large medical centers and teaching hospitals are used primarily for teaching purposes and are usually staffed with medical students and residents. Community hospital clinics, on the other hand, may be staffed by active attending physicians and are primarily for providing service. Since medical school enrollment is up dramatically over the last ten years, the need for teaching clinics is expected to continue. Generally, the service clinics have been more acceptable for patients than the teaching clinics.

The most interesting aspect of the outpatient component is the emergency department. Studies have shown that more than 60 percent of all emergency cases that visit emergency departments are not true clinical emergencies. This is a symptom of the problem of access and quality in our medical care system.

Why do so many patients use the emergency department? If we trace the evolution of the emergency department, we see that the volume began to increase sharply shortly after World War II, and it has continued to grow steadily since that time. The emergency departments remain the one marketplace of medical care where there is an interface between the middle class and the poor class. Both groups accept this service. There is no stigma in going to an emergency department. But there is definitely a stigma attached to waiting on a hard wooden bench in a teaching clinic of one of our urban medical centers.

There are very few financial barriers in going to the emergency department. They are open for emergencies and service and are not primarily interested in a patient's ability to pay. This is to the credit of the hospitals who sponsor them. It is not unusual to see a busy executive sitting next to a welfare recipient in a city emergency department. This is the one place in the outpatient component that has served to "bandage the gap" in the health care delivery system. But this is not enough.

Ambulance services are an outpatient activity that has taken on increased status with the advent of paramedics and the cardiopulmonary resuscitation teams. However, for millions who live in cities there are still two kinds of ambulance services. One is the municipal service, which is really an extension of the police ambulance or fire department. The other is the community ambulance staffed primarily for the people who can afford ambulances. This is another example of the two-class system.

An additional word about the clinics in our urban centers. These clinics are the embodiment of the two-class system. Many large teaching hospitals in urban centers find themselves serving a disproportionate number of poor and older citizens. Serious questions are being raised about the future of university teaching clinics. Many university medical centers and teaching hospitals are attempting to shift from staffing with medical students and residents to private practice and group practice arrangements. This is not an easy transition.

INPATIENT ELEMENT

The third element is the inpatient (hospital) component. This is characterized by the hospital bed. We have come to accept the hospital as synonymous with the bed. The number of hospital beds in short-term, nonfederal hospitals has increased to 980,000 from 505,000 in the 1950s. In this inpatient phase, Americans have asked the general hospital to provide a spectrum of care ranging from intensive to minimal. Hospitals continue to use the bed as the bench mark of occupancy, service, and financing, yet only 10 percent of the health needs of the patients in our system are cared for in the hospital.

The general hospitals in this country can be classified into two clinical groups: teaching hospitals and community hospitals. Despite a major overlap between the two groups, the major teaching hospital is a different species from the community hospital. Each group has its own needs and offers something different. Also, though both have inpatient beds and organizationally both have vertical and horizontal structures, their organizations are basically quite different. Time will tell which type of hospital has the most potential for change and improvement for the system.

The difficulties that are inherent in the hospital system stem from the dependency on the hospital bed. One model of the economy of hospitals indicates that hospitals are controlled by their medical staff who seek to maximize their own income and in so doing use the hospital bed extensively, which begins the vicious circle of increased hospital cost. As it now stands the economics of the hospital bed requires that the bed be filled for the hospital to stay solvent. The present inpatient system has a great deal of overlapping coverage. This is why mergers, shared services, and linkages are now in vogue and will undoubtedly increase and become more common. This trend may be one step toward improving care as well as toward holding a line on costs.

An interesting phenomenon in the inpatient system is that physicians are regarded by hospitals as both consumers and providers in the medical care arena. In this model, hospitals provide facilities not for the patient, but for the physicians who admit the patients. In turn, the physicians provide care to their patients and are therefore themselves providers. Understanding this arrangement is critical in identifying the control valve in the cost of medical care.

EXTENDED ELEMENT

The fourth element in the system is the extended component. Included in this area are such things as home care programs, skilled nursing facilities (SNFs), intermediate care facilities (ICFs), custodial care situations, boarding homes, visiting nurses, hospice care, and the like. Presently, less than 10 percent of the hospitals in this nation have home care programs. Is this sufficient? Do we need home care at all? Can home care really reduce our inpatient costs? If so, why aren't there more of them? Chronic hospitals are included in the extended element along with rehabilitation centers and other specialty hospitals and long-term care specialty hospitals. How many nursing homes are really needed? How does custodial care fit into nursing homes?

The scientific, professional component that has done such a magnificent job in our inpatient facilities seems to be lagging in the treatment provided in our skilled nursing facilities and in many of the other extended care programs. The extended component seems to receive very little support and therefore might deteriorate and become the weakest link in the system. As an illustration, one has only to look at the deplorable conditions of many of our nation's boarding homes.

COMMUNITY ELEMENT

The fifth and final element is noninstitutional. This is the community component. The community can be viewed from three perspectives. The first is a view of the community as a consumer group, those who use the health care facilities. Traditionally, consumers of hospital care have been a very passive group. The community consumer group includes health manpower resources, that is, the medical training programs in our medical schools and in our teaching hospitals. Aligned to this manpower element are the labor unions. Unions in this sense are seen not as third party payers but as representatives of manpower resources. They are a major force in the supply and demand function for labor. The second perspective embraces the community's consumers and their cultural situation as well as demographic shifts that affect our hospitals' long-range plans. This refers to the consumers and their ability to pay taxes and to the government's system of taxing that accounts for so much of our hospital reimbursement.

Finally, there is the perspective of the federal government as part of the community. In this context, we must consider the dollars that are spent on health care through the federal government. Americans spend 192.4 billion dollars on health care; that is 9.1 percent of the gross national product. Significantly, much of this expenditure comes through third party payers, including Medicare and Medicaid. Together, the Title XIX and Title XVIII programs account for 35.1 billion dollars in expenditures.

Apart from these aspects, the community element also includes the Blue Cross and Blue Shield Plans that have done such a great job in providing coverage for over 86 million Americans. Also included in this element are the results of legislation like the National Health Planning and Resources Development Act of 1974 and its recent 1979 amendment that have affected the system so dramatically. Beyond that, we would include in the community element the health educators and health environmental programs such as pollution control. Finally, in the community component we must include politics, the politics of health care.

From this examination, one thing is clear. If we in America are to move from a sickness care system to a true health care system, there must be more integration with the fifth element, the community. We must shift our concern away from the costly medical care components in the system. We must give impetus to education, proper recreation, successful employment, the concept of work, and to the psychological and social effects of human relations. Hard decisions must be made on what this country can afford to spend on medical care. If we are to move into a true health care system that works, we must come to grips with social goals and political goals, and with how they impact on the needs of a health care system.

NOTES

1. *Webster's New World Dictionary of the American Language, College Edition* (Cleveland and New York: The World Publishing Company, 1958), p. 1480.

2. James Haug and Kathleen Kuntzman, *Socio-Economic Factbook for Surgery 1979* (Chicago, Ill.: American College of Surgeons, 1979), p. 13.

Selected Hospital Occupations

Minimum Education Key

A. High School
B. Technical program or vocational school--two years or less
C. Two years of college, Associate degree
D. Four years of college, Bachelor's degree
E. Master's degree
F. Doctorate degree

Audiologist—An individual professionally trained and concerned with the assessment of hearing problems in adults and children. (D) For more information:

American Speech-Language-Hearing Association
10801 Rockville Pike
Rockville, Maryland 20852

Biomedical engineer—Concerned with the application of the biomedical specialty to the area of technology and methodology of medical equipment. (A) For more information:

Alliance for Engineering in Medicine and Biology
4405 East-West Highway, Suite 404
Bethesda, Maryland 20014

Biomedical equipment technician—Aids in maintaining, repairing, and operating the complex electronic biomedical equipment vital to the care and diagnosis of the patients in the hospital. (A) For more information:

Technical Education Research Center
44 Brattle Street
Cambridge, Massachusetts 02138

Blood bank technologist-MT (ASCP*) BB—Specialist in blood bank technology. Performs immunohematologic procedures. (C) For more information:

American Association of Blood Banks
30 North Michigan Avenue
Chicago, Illinois 60602

Certified laboratory assistant-CLA (ASCP)—Performs routine laboratory procedures. Works under the supervision of the medical technologist or pathologist. (B) For more information:

Board of Registry
American Society of Clinical Pathologists
P.O. Box 4872
Chicago, Illinois 60680

Cytotechnologist-CT (ASCP)—Works in the clinical laboratory. Stains, mounts, and screens microscopic slides for review by the pathologist. (C) (D) For more information:

American Society of Cytology
Health Sciences Center, Suite 1006
Thomas Jefferson University
130 South 9th Street
Philadelphia, Pennsylvania 19107

Dental assistant—Works with the dentist and dental hygienist in secretarial and clerical duties, in chairside assistance, and in certain laboratory work in the dental area. (B) (C) For more information:

American Dental Assistants Association
666 North Lake Shore Drive, Suite 1130
Chicago, Illinois 60611

Dental hygienist—Performs certain prophylactic dental treatments. Involved in teaching patients in dental care. (B) For more information:

American Dental Hygienist Association
211 East Chicago Avenue
Chicago, Illinois 60611

Dentist—A highly trained individual who treats diseases or injuries of the patient's teeth, jaw, and tissues around the teeth. (F) For more information:

American Dental Association
211 East Chicago Avenue
Chicago, Illinois 60611

---

*American Society of Clinical Pathologists

Dietician—Plans and directs the hospital food service, including the planning of meals and special diets, and directs the kitchen operations. (D) For more information:

The American Dietetic Association
430 North Michigan Avenue
Chicago, Illinois 60611

Electrocardiogram (EKG or ECG) technician—Works next to the patient, takes EKG readings that are interpreted by the cardiologist or other physician. (A) For more information:

American Cardiology Technologists' Association
Box 3425
Temple, Texas 76501

Electroencephalography (EEG) technologist—Operates the mechanical electrical device measuring electric activity of the brain; similar to the EKG technician with regard to heart readings. (A) For more information:

American Society of EEG Technologists
2997 Moon Lake Drive
West Bloomfield, Michigan 48033

Health educator—Relates to patients, indicating the importance of staying well and of preventive medical measures. (D) For more information:

Association for the Advancement of Health Education
1201 16th Street, N.W.
Washington, D.C. 20036

Histologic technician-HT (ASCP)—Cuts and processes microthin sections of body tissue for examination by the pathologists. (B) (C) For more information:

American Society for Medical Technologists
5555 W. Loop South, Suite 200
Bellaire, Texas 77401

Hospital accountant/controller—Works under the hospital controller involved in accounting activities in the hospital. (D) For more information:

Hospital Financial Management Association
666 North Lake Shore Drive, Suite 245
Chicago, Illinois 60611

Hospital administrator—The chief executive officer of the hospital who works with all aspects of hospital management, the board, and the medical staff. (E) For more information:

American College of Hospital Administrators
840 North Lake Shore Drive
Chicago, Illinois 60611

Hospital credit manager—Ascertains the patient's credit in using the hospital, is involved in collection activities of the hospital patient bills. (D) For more information:

Hospital Financial Management Association
666 North Lake Shore Drive, Suite 245
Chicago, Illinois 60611

Hospital engineer—Involved in providing lighting, plumbing and heating, and similar services for the hospital. (A) For more information:

American Society for Hospital Engineers
American Hospital Association
840 North Lake Shore Drive
Chicago, Illinois 60611

Hospital medical librarian—Provides an up-to-date library to meet the reference needs of students and personnel; provides stimulating recreational activities to all, including patients. (D) For more information:

Medical Library Association
919 North Michigan Street
Suite 3208
Chicago, Illinois 60611

Hospital personnel director—Responsible for hospital recruitment, selection, and placement of employees to fill staff vacancies; works closely with each hospital department head. (D) For more information:

American Society for Hospital Personnel Directors
American Hospital Association
666 North Lake Shore Drive
Chicago, Illinois 60611

Hospital public relations director—Works closely with the hospital administrator and staff; has responsibility for establishing the public relations and communications program within the hospital and hospital community. (D) For more information:

American Society for Hospital Public Relations Directors
American Hospital Association
666 North Lake Shore Drive
Chicago, Illinois 60611

Medical assistant—Performs a variety of clinical and administrative functions working for physicians. (B) For more information:

American Association of Medical Assistants
One East Wacker Drive, Suite 2110
Chicago, Illinois 60601

Medical laboratory technician-MLT (ASCP)—Performs a variety of clinical laboratory procedures under the direction of a qualified physician and pathologist or medical technologist. (C) For more information:

Board of Registry
American Society of Clinical Pathologists
Box 4872
Chicago, Illinois 60680

Medical record administrator—Head of medical records department; involved in the management, sorting, classifying, filing, and processing of medical records in the hospital. (D) For more information:

American Medical Records Association
875 North Michigan Avenue, Suite 1850
Chicago, Illinois 60611

Medical social worker—Deals with the patient's social, economic, personal, and community problems related to the patient's illness. (D) For more information:

National Association of Social Workers
2 Park Avenue
New York, New York 10016

Medical technologist-MT (ASCP)—Works in the hospital's clinical laboratory; involved in testing procedures in such areas as hematology, serology, and chemistry. (D) For more information:

Board of Registry
American Society of Clinical Pathologists
Box 4872
Chicago, Illinois 60680

Mental health technician—Works closely with and assists the other professionals in mental health activities dealing with emotionally disturbed and mentally retarded persons. (C) For more information:

National Association for Mental Health, Inc.
1800 North Kent Street
Arlington, Virginia 22209

Microbiologist —Works in large hospitals' clinical laboratory departments; involved in determining the structures of bacteria, viruses, and other organisms and in making cultures. (D) For more information:

> The American Institute of Biological Sciences
> 1401 Wilson Boulevard
> Arlington, Virginia 22209

Nuclear medicine technician and nuclear medicine technologist—Works in the nuclear medicine department under either the radiologist or the pathologist; works with radioactive isotopes that are administered to patients for diagnosis and treatment. (B or D) For more information:

> Society of Nuclear Medicine
> CNMT—Certified Nuclear Medicine Technologist
> 475 Park Avenue South
> New York, New York 10016

Nurse anesthetist—Member of the operating room team; a registered nurse with advanced training who works under the supervision of the anesthesiologist. (C) For more information:

> American Association of Nurse Anesthetists
> 216 West Higgins
> Park Ridge, Illinois 60068

Nurse-Licensed practical—Skilled in the care and treatment of patients in the clinical nursing unit; involved in most nursing tasks. (B) For more information:

> National League for Nursing
> 10 Columbus Circle
> New York, New York 10019

Nurse-Midwife—Registered nurse trained in the delivery of babies; works in both outpatient and prenatal setting and under the supervision of a physician in the delivery of babies in the hospital labor room and delivery suite. (E) For more information:

> American College of Nurse Midwives
> 1012 14th Street, N.W., Suite 801
> Washington, D.C. 20005

Nurse-Registered (RN)—Cares for patients in all clinical settings within the hospital. (C-D or Diploma) For more information:

> National League for Nursing
> 10 Columbus Circle
> New York, New York 10019

Nutritionist—Involved in the teaching of patients, both inpatients and outpatients, in various nutritional groups; may work in research and health surveys. (D) For more information:

> American Dietetic Association
> 620 North Michigan Avenue
> Chicago, Illinois 60611

Occupational therapist—Contributes to the physical and emotional rehabilitation of patients, using purposeful activities to teach new crafts or a vocation. (D) For more information:

> American Occupational Therapy Association
> 6000 Executive Boulevard, Suite 200
> Rockville, Maryland 20852

Operating room technician—Member of the surgical team, generally under the direct supervision of the operating room surgeon or a registered nurse. (A) For more information:

> Association of Operating Room Technicians
> 1101 West Littleton Boulevard
> Littleton, Colorado 80120

Pharmacist—Involved in dispensing and preparing drugs and medications; works closely with the medical staff and the nursing staff regarding pharmaceutical therapy. (D) For more information:

> American Association of Colleges of Pharmacy
> Office of Student Affairs
> 4630 Montgomery Avenue, Suite 201
> Bethesda, Maryland 20014

Physical therapist—Involved in modalities and rehabilitation of patients through physical therapy disciplines. (D) For more information:

> American Physical Therapy Association
> 1156 15th Street, N.W., Suite 500
> Washington, D.C. 20005

Physician—A graduate of a medical school or osteopathic school of medicine; involved in aspects of direct patient care and in the diagnosis and treatment of patients. (F) For more information:

> American Medical Association
> 535 North Dearborn Street
> Chicago, Illinois 60611

American Osteopathic Association
212 East Ohio Street
Chicago, Illinois 60611

Physician assistant—An individual who works under the direct supervision of a physician; assists physicians in patient care within their knowledge, skills, and abilities. (D) For more information:

Department of Allied Medical Professionals and Services
American Medical Association
535 West Dearborn Street
Chicago, Illinois 60610

Podiatrist—A professional involved in the diagnosis and treatment of ailments of the human foot, both medically and surgically. (F) For more information:

The American Podiatry Association
20 Chevy Chase Circle, N.W.
Washington, D.C. 20015

Radiation therapy technologist—Assists the radiologist in the treatment of disease and its effect by exposing the patient to x-ray or ionizing radiation under the direction of a radiologist. (B to D) For more information:

American Society of Radiologic Technologists
500 North Michigan Avenue, Suite 836
Chicago, Illinois 60611

Radiologic (x-ray) technologist—Member of the major staff component of the x-ray department; assists the radiologist in taking x-ray films and working with radiologic diagnostic activities in the department. (B to D) For more information:

American Society of Radiologic Technologists
500 North Michigan Avenue, Suite 836
Chicago, Illinois 60611

Recreational therapist—Involved in the rehabilitation of patients through therapeutic recreation; may be employed in specialty hospitals or larger hospitals. (D) For more information:

National Therapeutic Recreation Society
1601 North Kent Street
Arlington, Virginia 22209

Respiratory therapist—Administers breathing and diagnostic tests and provides therapeutic regimens and teaching to inpatients and outpatients. (B) For more information:

American Association of Respiratory Therapy
1720 Regal Row, Suite 112
Dallas, Texas 75235

Speech pathologist—Concerned with the treatment and assessment of speech disabilities in both children and adults; may work closely with ear, nose, and throat physician specialists. (D) For more information:

American Speech – Language – Hearing Association
10801 Rockville Pike
Rockville, Maryland 20852

NOTE

1. College of Allied Health Sciences, Thomas Jefferson University, *Health Careers Guidance Manual for the Greater Philadelphia Region* (Philadelphia, Pa.: Thomas Jefferson University, 1980).

Financial Statements

REVENUE AND EXPENSE STATEMENT

The revenue and expense statement identifies the hospital's major service functions and departments and compares their budget figures with their actual operating results. The simple statement of revenue and expenses (Exhibit B-1) provides an overall summary of the hospital's recent operating results and compares them with the month's budgeted figures. By reviewing this statement, management is quickly able to isolate changes in operating results. Other columns that might be included on such a statement are year-to-date, prior year-to-date, and budgeted figures.

BALANCE SHEET

The hospital's balance sheet (Exhibit B-2) provides a summary of what the hospital owns (its assets) and what it owes (its liabilities) on the last day of the hospital's accounting period. Each of the hospital's account balances has a specific and appropriate place on the balance sheet. The information contained on a balance sheet is restricted to financial data contained in the hospital's records. Additional information may be disclosed on the notes to the financial statements.

Exhibit B-1 ABC Hospital—Statement of Revenue and Expense
(Profit and Loss) for the Month of June

	Budget	Actual	Variance
Operating revenue			
Room and board	$270,000	$285,000	$15,000
Professional services	300,000	305,000	5,000
Other operating income	55,000	50,000	(5,000)
Gross operating revenue	625,000	640,000	15,000
Less: Allowances			
Contractual adjustments	65,000	70,000	5,000
Uncollectable (charity and			
bad debts)	20,000	25,000	5,000
Total allowances	85,000	95,000	10,000
Net operating revenue	540,000	545,000	5,000
Operating expenses			
Operating costs	80,000	90,000	10,000
Payroll costs	275,000	285,000	10,000
Depreciation	60,000	60,000	—
Interest	30,000	30,000	—
Total operating expense	445,000	465,000	20,000
Net gain from operations	95,000	80,000	(15,000)
Nonoperating revenue	10,000	10,000	—
Excess of revenue over			
expenses	105,000	90,000	(15,000)

Exhibit B-2 ABC Hospital Operating Fund: Balance Sheet—June 30, 19XX

Assets		Liabilities	
Current assets		Current liabilities	
Cash	$ 150,000	Notes payable	$ 200,000
Accounts receivable	1,900,000	Accounts payable	350,000
Less: Allowance for bad debts	(100,000)	Accrued expenses	80,000
Allowance for contractuals	(300,000)	Third party advances	200,000
		Current portion long-term debt	100,000
Net accounts receivable	$1,500,000	Total current liabilities	$ 930,000
Due to/from other funds	$ 50,000	Long-term debt	
Inventory	100,000	Mortgage payable	$3,900,000
Prepaid expenses	30,000	Leases	150,000
Total current assets	$1,830,000	Total long-term debt	$4,050,000
Property, buildings, and equipment		Total liabilities	$4,930,000
Land	$ 100,000		
Land improvements	80,000		
Buildings	7,000,000		
Fixed equipment	250,000		
Movable equipment	200,000		

Exhibit B-2 continued

Less: Accumulated depreciation	(3,000,000)	
Net property, bldg., and equip.	$4,630,000	
Fund balance		2,995,000
Other assets		
Board-designated assets	1,500,000	
Deposits	15,000	
Total other assets	1,515,000	
Total operating fund assets	$7,975,000	
Total liabilities and fund balance		$7,975,000

STATISTICAL REPORT

The data on a simplified statistical report (Exhibit B-3) shows the hospital's overall inpatient and key outpatient volumes. Because hospitals have such a high fixed cost complement, management must be sensitive to changes in service volumes. Accordingly, it is important to use this statistical data to analyze operating costs and operating revenue. For this purpose, it is common to display the hospital per-patient day costs and revenue amounts for a given accounting period.

A list of definitions relating to hospital financial statements is provided in Exhibit B-4. A brief list of definitions relating to operating statistics is presented in Exhibit B-5.

Exhibit B-3 ABC Hospital: Statistical Report for the Two Months Ended August 31, 19XX

	Current Month	Prior Month
Operating statistics		
Patient days	4,100	4,000
Maximum days per licensed capacity		
(150 beds)	4,500	4,500
% of occupancy	91%	89%
Average census	137	134
Average length of stay (for discharges)	7.5	7.3
Admissions	540	545
Emergency department visits	1,200	1,100
Outpatient visits	900	1,000
Per patient day		
Gross operating revenue	$156.00	$150.00
Total operating costs	$113.00	$110.00

Exhibit B-4 Definitions—Financial Statements

Accounts payable—Those obligations (bills) for goods and/or services the hospital owes that have not yet been paid.

Accounts receivable—An asset category that consists of full-rate charges to patients that are waiting to be settled (paid to the hospital). Usually found in hospitals where full-rate amounts are settled for less than full rates.

Accrued expenses—Expenses that the hospital has used or consumed through its operations but that have not been billed by the vendor; for example, salaries earned by employees but not yet paid to them.

Accumulated depreciation—Allowance for the depreciation account that contains the cumulative amount of depreciation taken on the various fixed assets. In hospitals, the allowance is generally calculated on the straight-line method.

Board designated assets—Unrestricted assets (funds) set aside by the board of trustees for specific purposes or projects.

Cash (operating fund)—The hospital asset, usually maintained in one or more bank accounts, for operating purposes. Cash in the form of contributions that are donor-restricted is accounted for differently and kept separate from unrestricted cash (operating) funds.

Contractual adjustments—This category is found on the Profit and Loss Statement and represents the difference between the hospital's full charge (rate) and the price (usually cost) that certain third party payers (e.g., Medicare) reimburse the hospital.

Contractual allowance—A Balance Sheet Account used to reduce gross third party accounts receivable to their realizable value.

Current liabilities—This is a category used to designate a hospital's obligation whose payment (liquidation) might reasonably be expected to use current assets. For example, a hospital could use cash to liquidate accounts payable.

Current position long-term debt—That portion of the long-term debt expected to be repaid within one year of the date of the financial statement.

Exhibit B-4 continued

Deposits—Funds set aside to insure the hospital's interest in a certain transaction (i.e., deposit on a leased parking lot).

Depreciation expense—The investment on the capital assets is allocated and recovered over the useful life of the assets. A depreciation factor is included in the hospital's charge structure and is generally considered an allowable cost by third party payers.

Due to from other funds—An asset or liability that is owed to or due from the operating fund of another hospital fund (i.e., plant fund). Such borrowings are referred to as interfund transactions.

Fund balance—The fund balance is what the hospital has left over in assets after the income and expenses have been handled.It is equivalent to the net worth category in an ordinary retail business balance sheet.

Gross operating revenue—The sum of all separate operating revenue accounts before any allowances or adjustments are removed.

Interest expense—The interest expense incurred on both capital and current indebtedness that is considered to be an allowable cost by third party payers.

Inventory—Goods in the hospital's possession such as medical/surgical supplies, drugs and medicines, office supplies, stationery, and forms.

Less: allowance for uncollectable—Reductions from gross operating revenue due to the medical indigence of the patient (charity or free care allowance), courtesy allowances (for clergy or medical staff), and bad debts.

Non-operating revenue—A revenue category that includes revenue not directly related to operating revenue, from patient care, patient services, or sale of related goods. The category includes unrestricted gifts and income (interest earned) from endowment funds.

Notes payable—Obligations incurred when the hospital issues its own note (promise) to secure a short-term loan from a bank or to postpone payment of an obligation to a vendor.

Exhibit B-4 continued

Operating costs—Includes the direct, indirect, and variable expenses incurred in operating functions of the hospital. Examples include supply expenses, purchased services, and fees to individuals and organizations.

Operating expenses—This is a heading commonly used in Profit and Loss Statements.

Operating revenue—Gross revenues earned at established hospital rates on an accrual basis.

Other operating revenue—Includes revenue from nonpatient care services to patients and sales to other persons such as visitors and staff. Examples include tuition paid for educational programs (such as nursing school) and sales of cafeteria meals to employees.

Payroll costs—Expenses for salaries, wages, and employee benefits.

Prepaid expenses—Expenses paid by the hospital but not yet used or consumed in hospital operations. Examples are insurance premiums paid in advance, interest paid in advance, and rentals of office machines paid in advance.

Professional services—A revenue category that includes revenue from the hospital ancillary services such as laboratory and x-ray and also includes revenue from special nursing areas such as operating rooms and central supply.

Property, buildings, and equipment—Asset category that includes the hospital's investment in land, buildings, and equipment used in hospital operations.

Room and board—A revenue category that may be called routine services or daily patient services. The category includes revenue from room, board, and general nursing services.

Third party advances—Monies paid to hospitals by third parties (e.g., Blue Cross, Medicare) against future services yet to be rendered and billed.

Total allowance—The sum of all separate allowance and adjustment categories.

Exhibit B-4 continued

Total current assets—The sum of all separate asset categories on the balance sheet.

Total current liabilities—The sum of all separate current liabilities categories.

Total liabilities—The sum of current and long-term liabilities of the hospital.

Exhibit B-5 Definitions—Operating Statistics

Admissions—The formal acceptance of an inpatient into the hospital. Inpatients are normally provided with room, board, and continuous nursing service and generally stay at least overnight.

Average census—The average number of inpatients presently in the hospital each day for a given period of time.

Average length of stay—The average number of days of hospitalization for inpatients who are discharged during the period under consideration. The average length of stay is calculated as follows:

$$\frac{\text{Total length of stay (discharge days)}}{\text{Total discharges}}$$

Emergency Department visit/outpatient visit—The visit of a patient to the hospital's emergency department or outpatient area located within the hospital proper or within facilities under the direction and sponsorship of the hospital.

Patient days—The unit of measure that denotes the services rendered to one patient over a 24-hour period.

Percent of occupancy—The ratio of the total inpatient service days for a period times 100 over the total inpatient bed count days for that same period.

Index

263

respiratory care, 111
social service, 163
volunteer, 152
hospital boards, 25
licensing, 210
medical staff, 70
education, 77
organization, 73
regulations, 75
outpatient care, 47
pharmacy, 116
physical medicine, 115
quality assurance, 194
social worker, 164
Joint Conference Committee, 77

K

Knights of St. John, 4

L

Labor
costs, 13, 14
Laundry Department
facilities, 127
linen control, 126, 127
support services, 126
Law
emergency department, 56-58
government health planning, 231, 232
medical records, 190
volunteers, 153, 154
Lazar Houses, 4
Leasing
purchasing systems, 139
Legal Implications. *See* Law
Liability
physicians' acts, 204
Licensing
history, 207
process, 210
Line Functions. *See* Functions
Linen. *See* Laundry Department
Linen Control
laundry, 126, 127

housekeeping department, 125
Location
departments
clinical laboratories, 102, 103
radiology, 107
Long, Crawford, 5
Long-Range Planning
agencies, 226
benefits, 229
committee, 227, 228
concept, 225, 226
contents, 229
history, 226, 227
laws, 231, 232
Long-Term Care Facilities
nursing services, 94

M

MacEachern, Malcolm, 162
Maintenance Department
biomedical equipment, 132, 133
energy conservation, 131
engineering, 130, 131
functions, 128
parking, 129
preventive maintenance, 128, 129
security, 130
staffing, 129, 130
Malpractice
costs, 203
defensive medicine, 203
liability, 204
magnitude, 201-203
Management
hospital
organization, 17-20
power, 21, 22
line vs. staff functions, 18
Marketing
concepts, 217, 218
hospital, 215
Medicaid, 6
emergency department, 55
generating revenue, 170, 171
Medical Care System. *See* Care; System

cyclical, 89
traditional, 89
special care units
coronary care, 92, 93
intensive care, 92
long-term, 94
nonacute, 93, 94
specialties
clinicians, 90
midwives, 91
practitioners, 90
staffing
case, 87
functional, 87
primary care, 88
team, 87
standards, 86
See also Nurses
Nursing Units
components, 83
floor plans, 84
services, 82, 83

O

Occupational Licensure
personnel department, 150, 151
See also Licensing
Occupational Safety and Health
Administration, 133
Occupations
education requirements, 243-251
O'Donovan, Thomas, 43
Organization
chart, 19
departments
anesthesia, 109, 110
clinical laboratories, 101
emergency, 51, 52
medical records, 188
nursing, 80, 82
radiology, 106
medical staff, 73, 74
power, 21, 22
pyramid, 17, 18
team of three, 18, 20, 21

See also Pyramid Organization
Orientation
volunteers, 153
Origins
hospitals, 3-7
nursing services, 79, 80
See also History
Outpatients
ambulatory surgery, 43, 44
clinics, 41-43
group practice, 45, 46
health care system, 237
medical office buildings, 44, 45
See also Inpatient
Outreach
health care system, 36
Outside Functions. *See* Functions

P

Parking Facilities
maintenance department, 129
Patient Stay
length of, 12
Patient Support Services
departments
dietary, 157-162
social service, 162-165
Patients
emergency department, 50
costs, 55
reasons, 51
rooms, 83
Patients' Bill of Rights, 62
Pathology Departments. *See* Clinical
Laboratories Department
Penn, William, 4
Pennsylvania Hospital of Philadelphia,
5, 6, 41
Personnel Department
fringe benefits, 145
function, 140
employment, 141-145
government involvement, 148-150
nurses, 145, 146
occupational licensure, 150, 151

Utilization Review
admitting department, 63
See also Professional Standards
Review Organization

V

Volume
emergency room, 50, 51
Voluntary Rotation
emergency department, 53
Volunteer Department. *See* Volunteers
Volunteers
administrative support services, 151
benefits, 154
director, 152, 153
ethics, 153, 154

Joint Committee on Accreditation of
Hospitals, 152
orientation, 153
role, 151
See also Director of Volunteers

W

Warwick Emergency Department, 59
Weber, Max, 17
Weed, Lawrence, 186
Wilmington General Hospital v.
Manlow, 59

X

X-Ray Department. *See* Radiology
Department

About the Author

I. DONALD SNOOK, JR., is the administrator at St. Mary Hospital in Philadelphia, Pennsylvania. Prior to assuming this position he was assistant director at the Thomas Jefferson University Hospital in Philadelphia. Mr. Snook has contributed numerous articles in the health care management literature. He holds an MBA in hospital administration from the George Washington University, a BS degree from the College of William and Mary, and a BBA in marketing from the Wharton School at the University of Pennsylvania. He has also completed the health management systems program at the Harvard Business School. Donald Snook is a faculty member in the graduate programs of health care administration at Temple University in Philadelphia and at Widener University in Chester, Pennsylvania.